People Throughout History Would Have Loved
Fit for Life Not Fat for Life . . .

"People who like this sort of thing will find this the sort of thing they like."

—**Abraham Lincoln**

"Life is not just being alive, but being well."

—**Martial**

"Every great advance in natural knowledge has involved absolute rejection of authority."

—**Thomas Huxley**

"All truth passes through three stages. First, it is ridiculed. Second, it is violently opposed. Third, it is accepted as self-evident."

—**Arthur Schopenhauer**

"Never allow schooling to interfere with your education."

—**Mark Twain**

D0051412

FIT FOR LIFE
NOT FAT
FOR LIFE

HARVEY DIAMOND

Coauthor of the
#1 *New York Times* Bestseller
Fit for Life

Health Communications, Inc.
Deerfield Beach, Florida

www.hcibooks.com
www.fitforlifetime.com

Library of Congress Cataloging-in-Publication Data

Diamond, Harvey, date.
    Fit for life not fat for life / Harvey Diamond.
       p. cm.
    Includes bibliographical references and index.
    ISBN 0-7573-0113-4
    1. Weight loss. 2. Reducing diets. 3. Nutrition. 4. Health.
    5. Raw food diet. I. Title.

    RM222.2.D482 2003
    613.2—dc21

                                      2003049971

Publisher: Health Communications, Inc.
           3201 S.W. 15th Street
           Deerfield Beach, FL 33442-8190

R-01-04

Cover design by Andrea Perrine Brower
Cover photo ©PhotoDisc
Inside book design by Lawna Patterson Oldfield

The body is a machine for living.
It is organized for that, it is its nature.
Let life go on in it, unhindered, and let it
defend itself. It will do more than if
you paralyze it by encumbering
it with remedies.

—Leo Tolstoy
War and Peace

CONTENTS

INTRODUCTION:
THE MIRACLE OF LIFE

Emblazoned across the front cover of *Newsweek* magazine, below a picture of a very obviously overweight child, the caption asks in large block letters:

"FAT FOR LIFE?"[1]

This book answers that question with a resounding no! Not *fat* for life—*fit* for life.

As I looked at the picture of this child on the cover of the magazine, a child so noticeably overweight, I could not help but be moved by his predicament. Certainly, he would much prefer to be singled out for a scholastic or athletic achievement, rather than for having to go to a "fat farm" to try to bring his weight under control. It is well established that if he does not figure out how to do so, not only will his childhood be riddled with health problems, but his adulthood as well.

Furthermore, I could not help but reflect on the problem of overweight that also continues to exist within the adult population. Nearly two-thirds of the American population is considered to be overweight to some degree. At any given moment, over 80 million people are said to be on special diets, spending billions of dollars every year on weight loss.

And I could not help but reflect on my own long-running and ongoing effort to keep my weight in check. I have been living on this planet for nearly sixty trips around the sun, and for my entire adult life, I have wrestled with my addiction to food and my desire to eat.

I cannot recall the number of times I have wondered, sometimes with amazement and sometimes with envy, how there can be people who can eat their own body weight in any kind of food they like, at any time of day or night, and not gain a single ounce, while others can put on five pounds merely by walking through the deli section of the grocery store. Those of us who dwell in the latter category know all too well that in order to maintain a reasonable body weight, we have to be ever-vigilant and diligent if we don't want to wind up blocking out the sun for those around us.

Except for programs that involve surgery and/or drugs, both of which I have an extreme aversion to, I have tried more weight-loss plans and "diets" than I care to recount. Not until I came to realize that there are certain fundamental truths that govern *all* human bodies—regardless of shape, size, genetic makeup or rate of metabolism—was I able to discover how to eat the foods I like and still keep my weight down.

These truths I refer to—you can call them laws, rules, principles or whatever you choose—*exist and are real.* And until they are acknowledged and respected, you can read all

500 or so diet books at your local bookstore; you can count calories, calculate grams of carbohydrates, fats and proteins, and measure portions; you can take appetite suppressants and starve yourself; you can drink powdered meal replacements and eat boring prepared diet foods that taste like straw; you can do all these things until the pyramids turn to dust, and it all will be to no avail. After all, aren't these the things people have been doing for years, even decades, and isn't the problem of overweight still as prevalent as ever?

The fact is, it doesn't matter if you are aware of the laws to which I am referring but choose to ignore them, or if you have never even been made aware of them: The end result will be the same. The effort to lose weight will be met with the same frustrations with which you are, in all probability, all too familiar.

Consider the law of gravity. No matter who you are, no matter if you are rich or poor, big or small, educated or not, male or female, and no matter where you live—be it in the United States, Asia, Africa or Europe—the law of gravity applies to all of us equally. Even if you don't believe in gravity, don't care for it and refuse to acknowledge it, if you don't respect it, the repercussions of violating it are the same. If a man falls, or even leaps, from a five-story building, he will be splattered on the ground, whether he is aware of the law of gravity or not. Someone might say, "Well, no wonder he's all smashed up. He broke the law of gravity." In actual fact, he didn't break the law of gravity; he *illustrated* it.

Other laws, equally as unyielding as the law of gravity, govern the human digestive tract and the process of eating food. Not being aware of them will not save you from the results of violating them. After reading this book, at least you will be aware of the principles to which I am referring, and you will be able to avoid the usual pitfalls and frustrations that customarily accompany attempts to lose weight.

You will be glad to learn how few of these truths there are, how marvelously easy they are to incorporate into your eating lifestyle, and how wonderfully simple it is to live in harmony with them, so that the eating experience remains a joyous one *while* you lose the weight you desire to lose.

There is no wealth but life.

—JOHN RUSKIN

What would you say is the one thing that is more precious to you or more valuable to you than anything else? Isn't it life? Glorious, magnificent, abundant life. How special and dear life is. All the money, all the diamonds, rubies, emeralds and sapphires, all the gold, all the riches the Earth can yield, all of it combined is but dust compared to a single moment of life.

The Hubble telescope is, by anyone's standards, an astounding conquest of science in action. It floats out in space taking pictures of stars, planets and galaxies that are billions upon billions of miles from Earth—so far away that we cannot even fathom the distances this remarkable piece of equipment manages to put before our eyes with crystal clarity.

What is it that differentiates our planet Earth from the billions of heavenly bodies that stretch out into the boundless expanse in every direction? Life. If the Hubble should happen to discover a single blade of grass a billion trillion miles from here, it would be heralded as the greatest, most monumental discovery of all time. And yet here we are on this tiny little orb floating out in the great void, and that little orb is teeming and bursting with life at every turn. It is a veritable island of prodigious superabundance—containing more life than all the rest of the known universe *combined.* How uniquely special and fortunate we all are to be here. What an indescribable gift life truly is. Yes, life is in a category all its own as it reigns supreme over all else.

As we look around at the limitless splendor and grandeur that is everywhere to be seen, it is impossible not to marvel at the incomprehensible intelligence that governs and directs all and everything that is life. Is it possible to think about these things and not simultaneously reflect on the nature of God? I don't think so. To me, it is impossible to think about or discuss life to any degree and exclude God from the process.

"Uh-oh," you may be saying, "looks like ol' Harv is drifting on me here. This is supposed to be a book on how to lose weight, and here he is talking about God. What gives?" My goal with this book is not only to show you how to shed unwanted weight from your body, but also to instill in you a brand-new reverence, admiration and respect for your body and the forces that preside over its well-being.

My desire is to write something that appeals to everyone and offends no one. That is a daunting challenge, even in

the best of circumstances. No matter what subject someone may write about—be it health, money, politics, relationships or whatever—he/she is bound to ruffle some
feathers somewhere along the line. Nowhere, it seems, is
that more so than when the subject of God comes up. So
I know I am treading on some delicate territory here. But
the plain fact is more people the world over believe in
some kind of God than do not. That means that in all likelihood, *you* believe in God. I would never, *ever* be so arro-
gant, bigheaded and foolhardy as to think I could tell you
what God is or how you should view God. What I *am* asking is that whenever I mention or say anything about God,
whatever is in your heart, mind and soul regarding your
own personal belief in God, see that. In no way is my aim
to push my beliefs about God on you or to try to change
your mind as to what your beliefs are or should be. But I
could no more discuss life and not mention God than I
could discuss the ocean and not mention water. There are
6.5 billion people on Earth, and that is precisely how many
valid, worthwhile and accurate depictions of God there
are. Call it God, the Grand Creator, Mother Nature, the
Almighty, the Life Force or any other term to which you
are partial. It is your own special, unique and personal
view of God that I'm asking you to bring to the fore and
reflect on.

God enters by a private door
into every individual.

—RALPH WALDO EMERSON

When I talk about the unparalleled intelligence that governs our lives down to the last, most infinitesimal detail, I am talking about God. Only God could figure out the mind-boggling intricacies that make life the grand spectacle it is.

There is an old saying that I absolutely love and have pondered more times than I can recall. It has been of great solace to me on numerous occasions. I have no idea where I first heard or read it; it's just one of those irresistibly captivating sayings that has been with me and has been the subject of contemplation for many years. "There is no place where God is not." I take this statement literally. There is not an event, situation or occurrence that is not God-directed. There is not a leaf that falls to the ground, not a song warbled in the throat of a songbird, not a flower that blooms and releases its scent, not a breath or step you or I take that is not touched by God's hand. And since God is, in my opinion, wholly loving and purely good, I am convinced that God did not drop us down on this planet, make us susceptible to every possible malady imaginable, not the least of which is obesity, and not also provide us with the means and ability to overcome any and all of it. God is more kind, loving and compassionate than that! No, in my mind God *wants* us to be happy, healthy and fulfilled, and has seen to it that whatever we need to be successful is here and available to us. The information you need to lose weight and keep it off while enjoying the eating experience and improving the overall health of your body exists. The question of the moment is, where is it and how do we find it? That, dear friends, is the subject of this book.

CHAPTER ONE

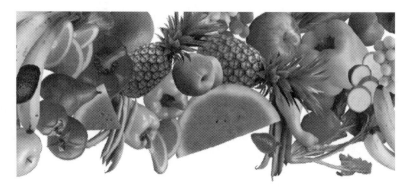

WHAT'S GOING ON HERE?

There's nothing new under the sun,
but there are lots of old things
we don't know.

—Ambrose Bierce

When I was in my late twenties back in the mid-1970s, I had already learned and put into practice with startling success the surprisingly simple tool that helped me lose, and keep off, the weight I had been wrestling with for years. Shortly, that very tool will be in your arsenal as well.

At that time I had been studying health and well-being for about four or five years, and because of the phenomenal success I had experienced, not only with weight loss, but also with other health problems I was facing, I was starting to have quite a high opinion of myself. Actually, I was a real know-it-all. Then, much to my great good fortune, I met and became friends with a gentleman in his eighties who brought me down to Earth. I think one of the very first things he ever said to me, which was only about a half-hour after we met, was, "You think you're pretty smart there, don't you, Sonny? Well, you don't know diddly." It took me a few weeks to get my ego in check enough to go back and talk to him some more. Thank heavens I did. After all, he was over eighty years old, was in tip-top shape, strong, witty, vibrant, sharp as a tack and "healthy as a horse." Ultimately, we took a real liking to one another, much to my benefit.

Mr. Bremmer lived in the mountains outside of Los Angeles, grew a good percentage of his own food and was truly one of the most outstanding people I have ever been fortunate enough to know. One of the reasons I loved hanging around Mr. Bremmer was that he was always dropping these little juicy tidbits of wisdom, and I learned a great deal from him during the time I knew him. Including, thankfully, some humility.

Now I'm in my late fifties, and I still recall with clarity many of the choice nuggets he imparted to me. One in particular stands out and is as true and relevant today as it was back then. We would be discussing some new breakthrough that was supposed to be the next great "miracle cure," which was instead proven to be just one more in a long procession of failures, and he would ask, "Why is it that people invariably try every incorrect remedy possible before relenting and trying the correct one?" That is the question that reverberates in my head whenever I reflect on the weight-loss industry in our country. And, oh, what an industry it is—an industry that generates astronomical profits for itself while leaving in its wake false hope, failures galore and a titanic junk heap of cast-off pills, potions and powders, devices of every type and design, and a countless number of temporary diets that offer such promise but ultimately deliver only disappointment.

In 1985 when the original *Fit for Life* was first published, the amount of money spent on weight loss in the United States was around $30 billion. Has it done any good? Is there less of a problem today than there was then? Have people figured out how to eat and still maintain a healthy weight? Has the weight-loss industry brought forth anything of lasting worth for the billions of dollars it has reaped? The answers to these questions are no, no, no and no. Today the money spent on weight loss is a mind-boggling $40 billion a year.[1] Good grief, that's over $100 million every day of the year—including weekends. Let's look at that figure with the full complement of zeros, shall we? It's $100,000,000 every single day.

Never in history has the situation been more dire. Not only are 60 percent of American adults overweight[2]—but, sadly, now even millions upon millions of children are also seriously overweight, and all indications are that it is becoming progressively worse both for adults and children. Why? I'll tell you why. Because people continue to allow themselves to try every incorrect remedy possible, instead of the ever-elusive correct one that is rooted in common sense, physiologically and biologically sound, and provides permanent results as a lifestyle, not some hit-or-miss scheme that is temporary at best.

Do you happen to know what a cashectomy is? Oh! You don't? Well, brace yourself, because whether you're aware of them or not, cashectomies are performed on you every day of your life with the precision of brain surgery. Most people have no idea whatsoever that cashectomies are being regularly performed on them. That's because cashectomies are so common in our society. They are going on everywhere, all the time. They are such an ingrained part of the very cell structure of our culture that precious few people even have a clue as to what's being perpetrated against them. They are simply viewed as the normal, natural process of commerce.

> *Advertising may be described as the science of arresting the human intelligence long enough to get money from it.*
>
> —Stephen Leacock

Here's the definition of a first-rate cashectomy: the process of convincing you to hand over fat fistfuls of your hard-earned cash for a product or service you are convinced will in some way improve your life and well-being, but receiving instead something that hurts you, makes you sick or kills you.

My friends, there are experts in the field of cashectomology who have you permanently fixed in their crosshairs. They work day and night to figure out new and innovative ways to get you to unload the contents of your purse or wallet for something worse than worthless— something harmful or life-threatening. They are hard at work this very moment, and *you* are the object of their efforts. Brothers and sisters, listen, and listen well. Any time $100,000,000 is tossed around *every single day*, the professional cashectomists are going to be climbing all over one another to get their piece of the pie. And for the cashectomists plying their trade in the weight-loss industry, no scheme, ploy, ruse or subterfuge is off-limits in trying to separate you from your cash. Or as George Gurdjieff put it, "To milk you of your oof."[3] Whatever they have to do to cajole, entice and ensnare you, they will. Sounds heartless and cold, I know, but it is high time the truth be told. Those who are desperate to lose weight *will* be preyed upon with one of the three D's: a diet, a device or a drug.

1. **DIETS.** The first chapter in the first *Fit for Life* book ever published was entitled "Diets Don't Work." Here it is nearly twenty years later, and I'm saying it again: *Diets don't work!* They are temporary measures that reap temporary results. Do you want to be temporarily rich? Do you want to be temporarily in love? Do you want to be temporarily healthy? No? Then why temporary weight loss? Is it fun taking off weight only to put it back on and then repeat the cycle? Do you like measuring portions, counting calories, being deprived and taking the joy out of the eating experience? Of course not. I know that. And you will never have to again once you have learned the ageless secret of success that renders diets obsolete, which I will reveal to you in the next chapter.

2. **DEVICES.** There are no devices that will magically take weight off your body. Do you remember those ab machines that used to be for sale? They promised that all you had to do was attach some electrodes to your body and sit around and watch TV, while the machines magically gave you a washboard stomach. So absurd was the idea that the government had to step in and put a halt to the sham, but not before millions of dollars were made for the cashectomists who I'm sure were high-fiving one another as they danced all the way to the bank.

We put drugs of which we know little,
into bodies of which we know less,
to cure disease of which we
know nothing at all.

—Voltaire

---

3. **DRUGS.** The cruelest of the cruel. It's one thing for
a diet or a device to not fulfill its promised results. It's
frustrating and annoying to put in effort with no
reward. But drugs can *kill* you. We live in a fast-food,
quick-fix world where we want what we want, and we
want it right now! Those who push drugs for a living
prey on that mentality.

Whether it's Fen-Phen, Meridia or any number of other
pharmaceuticals that come on the scene amidst proclamations of being the latest "miracle cure" for weight loss, only
to be found to be deadly and then withdrawn from the
market, all drugs are poisons. *All!* There isn't one that does
not have side effects. A student in medical school takes
numerous classes on toxicology. Do you know the meaning
of the word *toxicology?* The study of poisons. These drugs
make billions of dollars for the cashectomists before it's
revealed that they kill people, only to be replaced by the
next one in line.

Unfortunately, drugs have become a way of life in this
country. You can no longer turn on the TV without being
deluged with slick, expensively made commercials that go

over the top in extolling the possible benefits while minimizing the possible harm. Law requires that a drug commercial has to list the *most common* side effects, so the most destructive needn't be mentioned. It's one thing to hear "the most common side effects are headaches, nausea and abdominal pain." As unappealing as that is, what if you heard, "can cause angina, liver failure and death"? You wouldn't be so quick to pop those pills then, would you?

> More die of the remedy
> than of the malady.
>
> —FRENCH SAYING

Here's a little tidbit you may not be aware of. Did you know that every year 2 million Americans become seriously ill and 106,000 die from prescription drugs?[4] The study bringing this to light clearly states that the cause of illness and death is from "toxic reactions to correctly prescribed medicines taken properly." These are not accidents or overdoses or the improper mixing of different drugs. These deaths are from taking the *correct* drug, in the *correct* dose, at the *correct* time, in the *correct* way. In other words, taking drugs in the exact proper way they were intended to be taken kills more people every year than breast cancer, prostate cancer and AIDS combined. And guess how these deaths are classified? No, they're not simply called "deaths" just because that's what they are. That's too cold and harsh. They're referred to as "adverse drug events."[5] Ah, yes, that's so much more genteel. So let's say, for example, that you succumb to one of the advertisements for a prescription appetite suppressant, and after taking it for a while you become violently sick and are taken to the hospital. Your loved one could show up to check on you and be told, "Oh, he/she's had an adverse drug event."

"Really, well, how adverse was it?"

"He/she's dead."

I don't mean to be flippant or callous here, but what I'm telling you is *real*, and looking the other way is not going to serve you very well.

What I find to be most lamentable about the $40 billion spent each year—whether it's for some regimented, temporary program; surgery to make someone's stomach smaller; meal-replacement drinks; or drugs that can kill—is that none of these measures address the problem at the core. None remove the *cause* of overweight. And that suits the weight-loss industry just fine. After all, the only way to make another $40 billion next year, and the year after that, is if people remain overweight. If the cause of overweight were to be understood and eliminated, look at all that lost income.

Do you know why the people making billions of dollars at casinos in Las Vegas and Atlantic City don't hold classes teaching the public how to beat the house? It's the same reason why the weight-loss industry is not particularly interested in your learning how to lose weight and keep it off, or how to avoid becoming overweight in the first place. It's one thing to gamble and lose money. It's something altogether different to gamble and lose your life, don't you think?

I'm not going to bore you with the long list of statistics around the problem of obesity; you wouldn't be reading this book if you weren't already familiar with a good number of them. But a few are worth mentioning.

What did you do today? Did you go to work, play with your kids, spend time with a loved one, walk in the park, read a book, exercise, watch a sunset, enjoy a meal with a friend, sit and marvel at the world around you and thank God for the gift of life? All these activities and more are available to you every day. Let me tell you what more than 800 people in the United States did today. They died[6]—as a result of obesity. And more than 800 died yesterday, and the day before that, and more than 800 will die tomorrow and the day after that. Every day, 365 days a year, more than 800 people die—300,000 a year. Most of these deaths are from cardiovascular causes. The heart can't take the extra weight.

As regards other causes, obese individuals have a 50 to 100 percent increased risk of death from *all* causes, compared with normal-weight individuals.[7] In the 1990s, obesity increased in every state in the United States in both genders and across all races/ethnicities, age groups, educational levels and smoking statuses.[8] Recently the World Health Organization stated that obesity has reached such epidemic proportions that world health officials have decided that they need to take a more aggressive approach if they are to head off a global explosion of fat-related diseases.[9]

In the largest and most comprehensive study of its kind ever conducted, reported in the *New England Journal of Medicine*, more than 90,000 cancer deaths per year could be prevented by losing weight. The study reflects a tenfold increase from the largest previous study (900,000 people studied over a sixteen-year period). One reaearcher stated, "Because of the magnitude and strength of the study, it's irrefutable, it's absolutely convincing."[10]

We've heard these ominous reports in the past, but the one factor that is different now, indeed the factor that sends home the message more than any other that the situation has reached a critical state unlike any other time in history, is the degree to which children are overweight or obese. It is estimated that 22 million of the world's children *under five* are overweight or obese.[11] Here in the United States, where we take such pride in being a beacon of inspiration in all areas of life, the prevalence of overweight children is a national disgrace. The number of overweight children in the 1990s more than doubled, in fact nearly tripled, since the 1960s and 1970s.[12]

I'd say the time has come for us to get serious and rededicate ourselves in a direction that actually produces some long-term results. How about you? How much proof is needed to see that the entirety of what has been attempted to date has failed? Not only has the situation gotten progressively worse year after year, decade after decade, for adults, but now, as a result of the choices made over the years, our children are being forced to deal with the consequences of those nonproductive decisions.

Common sense is very uncommon.

—Horace Greeley

Nothing could possibly be more obvious than the fact that something brand-new is needed. An entirely new and different approach is called for. It is time for a voice of reason and common sense to rule the day as regards the challenge of losing weight, comfortably, intelligently and permanently. We're not just talking about dropping a few pounds so we can fit into our bathing suits for summer. *The crisis has now filtered down to our children.* Nothing will ever convince me that this is what the Grand Creator intended for us. It is time to shut the door on the mistakes of the past. No more mindless crash diets that fly in the face of reason. No more "seventy-two-hour wonder diets" or "four-week miracle cures." No more tummy tucks, liposuction, stomach stapling or other surgical procedures that attack the symptom while ignoring the cause. No more toxic drugs that poison the body and put life at risk. *No more!* All of the incorrect remedies have been fully explored over and over, and time has proven them all to be ineffectual. It is now time to embrace the correct remedy—the one that is in alignment with life, is based in common sense, resounds with logic and reason, and definitely proves its own worthwhileness.

There is a gigantic, mind-numbing irony in all of this— an irony so striking there are not words to describe it in the dictionary. As millions of people chase after outlandish, unrealistic remedies that have failure built right into them, spending fortunes on them only to find out they have been taken on a fanciful, promise-laden road to nowhere, the simple solution to the problem of overweight sits like a shining jewel, unnoticed, unutilized and unfulfilled right before our eyes. Irony of ironies.

The challenge facing me now is not how to organize the information you yearn for into a cohesive program that reaps results. Nor is the challenge for me to be able to relate the information to you in a comprehensive fashion that will be easily understood. Frankly, that's the easy part. The solution is literally so simple, obvious and straightforward that it just cannot be denied by any fair-minded person willing to give it a fair hearing.

It is actually the simplicity of the message that may elude you, not the grasping of it. Remember my friend Mr. Bremmer lamenting that he wondered why people try all the incorrect methods before settling on the correct ones? Well, I think I know why. It's because the correct remedy is *too* simple and obvious. I know how ridiculous that must sound, but I'm serious. And that is the task that lies before me: to overcome the mind-set, the belief system that the gargantuan problem of overweight that affects too many millions of people and costs so many billions of dollars could actually be remedied by something totally uncomplicated, practical and accessible.

No statement should be believed
merely because it has been
made by an authority.

—HANS REICHENBACH

People have been systematically convinced that there are no easy answers, so that becomes their reality. This way of thinking is supported and solidified by the scientific community. There is no shortage of so-called experts in the field who are constantly offering up the latest theories. All manner of conjecture, supposition and speculation are put forth by reasonable-sounding, highly credentialed authorities who differ completely with other reasonable-sounding, highly credentialed authorities, so the beleaguered seeker in the middle is bounced around like a tennis ball, not knowing what to think or what to do.

If it's not some gene that is deemed to be the culprit in putting on weight, it's some newly discovered appetite-boosting hormone secreted by the stomach.[13] Or it's some other impossibly complicated, jargon-laden theory that no one except those who spend their days filling and emptying beakers and petri dishes in a laboratory can understand. The explanation invariably ends up with the same tired old refrain of "a lot more research will have to be done before we can . . . blah blah blah blah. . . ." It then regularly ends up with "hopefully there will be a new drug in the next few years."

If it's *not* on the molecular level, then it's what body type you are or emotional type you are or blood type you are. It's all lots of graphs and charts, height and weight distinctions, categories and groups, all designed to pigeonhole you into just the right classification so you can know what your jumping-off point is in the grand battle against the always-advancing enemy that is bound and determined to make your clothes too tight.

After years and years of the same old stuff that never ever brings anything forth that works and is lasting; after trying the latest breakthrough with great resolve only to have your efforts dashed on the rocks of disappointment; after failure piled on top of failure—I can see where my contention that the solution to the entire mess is as simple and straightforward as falling off a log might be met with some skepticism.

When you think of the strongest animals on Earth, which do you perceive to be the very strongest of all? Most people rightly name the elephant and, aside from some whales, the elephant is also the largest. These impressive beasts can stand over ten feet tall and weigh more than 12,000 pounds. The largest-known elephant measured over thirteen feet tall and weighed more than twelve tons! Elephants can perform phenomenal feats of strength, carrying cargos of 600 pounds with ease or moving logs that weigh up to two tons. When lions were proclaimed "King of the Jungle," there must have been a weight and size restriction to enter the running, for elephants are truly the masters of the animal kingdom in terms of size and sheer power. An enraged elephant on a full run can strike fear into the heart of *any* animal in its path.

Elephants in India have been used extensively for centuries to perform heavy tasks after they are tamed and trained. The process of taming begins at a young age when they are shackled to huge trees with very heavy iron chains. No matter how hard the young elephant tries to break away, it can't. Finally, it gives up trying. As soon as it reaches the full length of its chain, it simply stops right there and makes no other attempt to go further. As time goes by, both the size of the tree and the strength of the chains are decreased until the elephant cannot escape from even a flimsy little rope tied to a small branch. Having grown up with the inability to wander further than the length of its restraints, the moment the elephant feels resistance upon its leg, it stops, thinking it can go no further. Even though it could easily pull away from the flimsy rope that has it tethered to a peg in the ground, it has been convinced that it does not have the power to do so, and so it remains captive even though it could easily go anywhere it wanted whenever it pleased.

Whatever, pray tell, could all this have to do with the subject at hand? Good question. I can't help but compare the plight of the elephant, which, although possessing extraordinary power and strength, is effectively subdued, to the plight of those seeking to lose weight. The elephant's belief system is that it can't move beyond the length of its tether. The weight-loss seeker's belief system is that the answer to successful, long-term weight loss cannot be simple. Both are mistaken.

Never underestimate your power
to change yourself.

—H. JACKSON BROWN JR.

I have long been labeled an idealist. I've worn that label as a badge of honor. I pride myself on always expecting the very best of everyone. However, I am also a realist, especially in matters such as the content of this book. The idealist in me wants to think that anyone who has ever struggled with his or her weight, be it with ten pounds or fifty pounds, will, upon learning the simple message this book imparts, rejoice at discovering the long-awaited answer and immediately put into practice the newfound information. The realist in me knows better.

The plain fact is that regardless of how sensible and promising this book or any other book on the subject is, it will only appeal to some and not to others. That's just how things are. Permit me to help you clarify which category you are in. If you are hoping to find within these pages a temporary, quick-fix dietary regimen that is adhered to for a while until you drop the desired weight, only to return to the same old habits that made you overweight in the first place, I can tell you right now this book is definitely not for you. Or if you are hoping for a breakthrough pill or potion that will magically do for you what only a sensible, logical and reasonable effort on your part will achieve, again, you will find nothing like that here.

You can't cross the sea merely
by standing and staring at the water.
Don't let yourself indulge in vain wishes.

—SIR RABINDRANATH TAGORE

However, if you are one of those people who have had your share of disappointments and are fed up with riding the merry-go-round of yo-yo diets that promise everything and deliver nothing of permanence; if you genuinely want to finally, mercifully, learn a permanent, lifelong eating lifestyle that allows the eating experience to remain a joyous one (not a clinical endeavor of denial and frustration) that proves itself with visible, clearly defined results and is remarkably easy to grasp and implement, and so uncomplicated and forthright that you can confidently explain it to anyone, even a child—then this will be your Holy Grail.

As an ex-pudgy myself, I have tried more diets and schemes than I care to recall. So I want you to know that I completely understand if you are reading this and experience just a tad of skepticism. If you're anything like me, you've heard assurances similar to the ones I am making, charged headlong into a new approach with great resolve, only to find out that it wasn't as simple or obvious as promised.

All I can tell you is that *this* time you are going to be pleasantly surprised because you are about to see the truth of what I've been saying about its simplicity. Many times in situations like this you're told you only have to follow "six simple steps" or only "three simple steps" to be successful. Well, guess how many simple steps you will be called upon to follow through on here? One! Yes, that's right, one! It can't be simpler than that, can it? No joke, there is only *one* concept for you to grasp. Only *one* action to take, and the problem of overweight will become a thing of the past.

Have I aroused your curiosity? Well, turn the page, and let's get right to it.

CHAPTER TWO

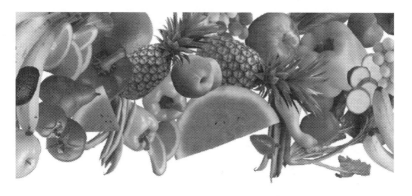

LIVING OR DEAD?
YOU CHOOSE

That greatest miracle of all,
the human being.

—MARYA MANNES

Do you recall that this book started with me praising the magnificence of life? Therein lies the secret of success. You're looking for a miracle? *You* are a miracle. The life that animates every cell in your body is a miracle, the grandest miracle of all.

Nothing could be more elemental and more self-evident than the statement, "Life begets life, and death begets death." You might be saying, "Gee, no kidding. Tell me something I don't know." But as obvious and brimming with truth as that statement is, there are those who have allowed themselves through advertising, propaganda and conditioning to lose sight of that simple truth.

Everything that lives is holy,
life delights in life.

—WILLIAM BLAKE

What if I posed the title of this chapter to you in the form of a question: "Living or dead, what's your choice?" It's almost laughable to think anyone would choose death over life in *any* circumstance. Whether you are consciously aware of it or not, you are called upon to make that choice every single day, and you might be shocked to learn what your decision is more often than not.

Whatever could I be talking about? I am referring to your food choices. What are our most urgent necessities for life? Air, water and food. We have scant, if any, control over the air we breathe, not that it's air that makes us fat. We are water beings living on a water planet. Both our bodies and the surface of Earth are approximately 70 percent water. We have far more control over the type and quality of water we drink, and we must be diligent in seeking out the purest available. But, again, it's not the water we drink that makes us fat. So, what is it? Let's see . . . what's left? Oh yeah, *food!* We will each eat approximately seventy tons of food in our lifetimes, and it is the quality of that food that will be the greatest determining factor in the quality of our lives—the greatest determining factor in whether we will be overweight or not.

Remove any one of the three primary necessities of life and we die. Without air, life will end in about six minutes. Without water, life can go as long as two to three weeks, although most would succumb in about a week to ten days. Without food, death would occur in about six to eight weeks, although there are extraordinary cases of people surviving longer. One thing is for certain: Depriving the human body of food will result in death. We've all heard the old saying, "You are what you eat." A truer statement has never been uttered.

The living human body is made up of living cells. Lots of them. I've heard estimates ranging from 75 to 125 trillion cells. Each and every cell is bursting with life. Seen under a microscope, a single cell bustles with unimaginable activity. Tens of thousands of chemical actions and reactions take place every moment, taking in nutrients, performing the activities of life and eliminating waste. Every day approximately 300 billion cells die off and are replaced by living ones that are produced at the impressive rate of about 200 million every minute.[1] Guess what the new replacement cells are made from? *The food you eat.* It is an absolute, unassailable fact that our bodies are made of the food we eat, and if food is withheld, we die. This isn't conjecture. This isn't open for debate. No food, no life.

We come now to the very heart of the matter—the heart of this book. The health and the *weight* of your body are entirely based on the type and quality of the food you eat. So here it is my friends: the simple, obvious, straight-forward answer to the problem of overweight that I have been alluding to. It is the one concept you need to grasp and the one action you need to take to end the battle for the rest of your life. Don't blink because it can be revealed in its entirety with one short sentence, which appears in bold to the right.

EAT MORE LIVING FOOD THAN DEAD FOOD!

That's it. That is the corner-stone of this book, and everything else is merely commentary.

Now that I've stated it, after all the build-up, I can understand if you are a bit unsatisfied. Perhaps you were expecting it to be something more esoteric or momentous. Questions may be coming to the surface such as, "Oh, come on, man, that's all you have to tell me?" Or, "What in blazes does he even mean by that?" Or, "Huh?" But remember, I have told you all along it is so uncomplicated and straightforward that the simplicity of the message is what has eluded people. If you *are* feeling at all let down, yes, I want you to know that I understand because no matter how much I tried to prepare you for the fact that it was something astonishingly simple, I think the tendency is still to expect something super-extraordinary that would blow your mind—some totally unexpected revelation that would magically, miraculously ring true like nothing else ever had before.

I am asking you to please hang in there with me—you won't be sorry. I have been familiar with, worked with and seen the results of people eating more living food than dead food for nearly thirty-five years. You have had but a few moments to give thought to and contemplate the concept. I want to assure you that the more familiar you become with it, the longer you have to ponder it and, most importantly, the longer you have actually incorporated it into your lifestyle, the more it will reveal itself to be the momentous and extraordinary concept it is.

All great ideas are controversial,
or have been at one time.

—George Seldes

I promise you that by the time you have finished the book, you will have a brand-new understanding and appreciation for what eating more living food than dead food means. And all questions and concerns you may have now as to how doing so will help you lose weight will be answered.

If you desired to play the piano, it is extremely unlikely that you would realistically think that after learning all the keys and taking a couple of lessons you would be ready to give a concert at Carnegie Hall. If you want to become good at something, you have to practice it—whether it's playing the piano, operating a computer or riding a bicycle. It's the same thing here. As I stated earlier, you have just learned of the concept of eating more living food than dead food so you understandably have no familiarity with it. Over the course of this book, that will change.

Everything you need to know about what living and dead foods are, why it is important to eat more living than dead food, what can be expected upon doing so, and how to intelligently and comfortably incorporate more living food than dead food into your eating lifestyle will be revealed in detailed, unencumbered plain talk. Then, after seeing the wisdom of the concept itself, it will just be a matter of experiencing firsthand the results that automatically ensue once the principle is put into practice.

The first step in this process is to define what living foods are and what dead foods are. Twenty years ago, prior to the release of the original *Fit for Life*, I counseled people one-on-one. They felt sick or couldn't take off the weight they desired, so I would familiarize myself with their personal dietary background and then design a personalized program for them to follow in order to achieve their goals. This played a huge role in my own education and understanding of the relationship between diet and health. I was then and am today astounded at how few people can describe the difference between a food that is living and a food that is dead.

Usually the first thing that would come to mind when they thought of a dead food was some kind of meat because an animal had to die to provide it. "You mean like a hamburger or something?" It's amazing how oriented we are to eating meat in this country. You'd be stunned to know how many people, upon my asking them how much living food they ate, would ask, "You mean like raw meat or fish?"

The very first thing I would ask of those who came to me for advice was to describe to me what their diet was, not in generalities but in meticulous detail. Then I would ask them to describe what they put into their bodies on one average day, leaving out absolutely nothing no matter how small an amount. I can't recall a single instance where those I was helping were not shocked and dismayed, nearly to the point of embarrassment, upon learning the huge disparity of living food over dead food that predominated their diets. It turned out to be about 10 percent living. Occasionally it was more, but with more frequency it was less. Of course, that was precisely why they were seeking my help.

The easiest way for me to explain the difference between living food and dead food, so that there can be no possible mistake in your understanding, is by explaining what enzymes are. More and more as of late, enzymes are being researched and talked about with increasing regularity, and with good reason. Perhaps you have been hearing about them yourself but aren't quite sure exactly what they are or, more importantly, what an immense and immeasurable role they play in our lives.

We cannot help but be impressed with the profusion and diversity of life that is abundantly displayed at every turn. This little jewel of a planet is bursting with more life than all of the rest of the known universe combined. If it were not for enzymes the planet Earth would be as lifeless as the moon or Mars. Literally. Every plant, every animal, every human being lives because of enzymes. The animating force or power or principle that allows life to be lived resides inside these tiny little protein chemicals called enzymes.

A living food is, therefore, one that has its enzymes intact. A dead food is one that has its enzymes destroyed. It's as simple as that. And how are enzymes destroyed? *Heat!* At the temperature of 118°F, enzymes are wiped out. I don't mean they are compromised or degraded—they are obliterated. And 118°F is far, *far* less heat than is required to cook food.

If you are anything like the people I described above, whom I counseled one-on-one, and if you are still struggling to bring your weight down to a more comfortable level, chances are you are not eating nearly the amount of living food you should be eating. If your diet is most heavily dominated by foods that are devitalized and denatured, in other words, dead, then you are only making your effort more difficult. Ever hear of Sisyphus? In Greco-Roman mythology Sisyphus was doomed to forever push a huge, heavy stone uphill. If he ever stopped pushing it up, it would roll back down, and he would have to start all over again. Attempting to successfully and permanently lose weight while trying to nourish the living body with more dead food than living food is to put yourself in the same predicament as the ill-fated Sisyphus.

We never stop investigating.
We are never satisfied that we know
enough to get by. Every question we
answer leads on to another question.
This has become the greatest
survival trick of our species.

—DESMOND MORRIS

It's very interesting to me how human beings take such pride in being able to solve the most complicated and challenging problems, to take on tasks of monumental difficulty and adversity and come out victorious. Any apparently insurmountable, mazelike enigma, the more puzzling and baffling the better, is taken on with an indomitable resolve, with an Einstein-like perseverance until people triumph and the solution is achieved. Anything from the making of a computer chip to constructing a rocket ship to go to the moon—nothing is beyond our ability to prevail. Except, it seems, figuring out how to eat so as not to become overweight.

What I find to be equally interesting are those people who delight in unraveling the most complex and obscure of concepts but are somehow incapable of grasping the simplest ones. Those people who are overeducated or educated beyond their intelligence seem to be convinced that there are no simple answers to difficult questions. And nowhere is that way of thinking more prevalent than when discussing the enormous benefits that can be realized by the simple action of eating more living food than dead food.

"Surely it can't be that simple or we would already have discovered it." We have been told for so long that the problem of overweight is a daunting challenge that is far too complex for there to be any simple answers that most people, especially those who have "tried every diet that has come down the pike," have come to believe it. So much so that I have actually known people to *complain* that it's too simple to accept. I then have to ask them, "If the answer were something more complicated, more inconvenient and more expensive, would you have more faith in it then?"

Your understanding of how to lose weight successfully comes down to your acknowledging the truth behind the statement, *living bodies require living food*. It seems ludicrous, almost comical that something so obvious would even have to be stated.

Instead, I feel like I need to repeat it at least a dozen times and shout it out at the top of my voice:

LIVING BODIES REQUIRE LIVING FOOD!

We humans stand alone as the one and only species on Earth to cook all the life out of our food before eating it and then wonder in dismay why we don't feel well and can't lose weight. The only time other animals, the so-called "lower animals," become overweight is when they come into contact with us. Wild dogs and wild cats never, *ever* become overweight. But let them become our pets and eat food that has had all the life cooked and processed out of it, and you start to see dogs and cats become pudgy.

If it is indeed true that living food is so very much more important to eat than dead food, we might understandably wonder how and why we ever started eating cooked food in the first place. I have pondered that very question myself. Who knows for sure? It certainly must have had something to do with the discovery of fire. Long before prehistoric civilizations had emerged from the Stone Age, our ancestors must have been introduced to fire as the result of naturally occurring blazes that wiped out everything in their path. We can only imagine what it was like for those who witnessed fire for the first time. Perhaps coming upon an animal that had been "roasted," a hunter took a hunk and ate it and said to his friend, "Hey Ug, try this." And from that day, when everything eaten was uncooked, thereby alive, to this day, we have been sealing our fate by eating more and more cooked food—to the point where only a very small percentage of what we eat today is alive.

There is one thing stronger than
all the armies in the world, and that is
an idea whose time has come.

—Victor Hugo

For the complete, clearly stated message of how to recapture control of your life as regards your health and your weight, which are as inseparable as a tree is to the ground on which it stands, read the words in bold at the right.

SINCE LIVING BODIES REQUIRE LIVING FOOD, EAT MORE LIVING FOOD THAN DEAD FOOD.

We couldn't hope for a more no-nonsense, straight-forward premise to live by than that.

As you progress through this book, it will become entirely clear to you exactly what I mean by "living food." For now, I wish to allay any concerns you may have that I will be suggesting you eat raw meat. Considering the number of different bacteria that can thrive on raw meat, and the fact that some of them can be deadly, I would never recommend eating raw meat of any kind. In truth, it is a practice that definitely should be avoided. As you will soon learn, living food refers primarily to fruits and vegetables in their natural, uncooked state.

Now, we would never dream of putting the incorrect fuel in our cars. To put Coca-Cola or water in the gas tank instead of gasoline would be viewed as lunacy by most everyone. But for some inexplicable reason, that is exactly what we are doing to our bodies. The living body can no more function properly on dead food than a car can run on Coca-Cola. Just as you know very well that you have to put gasoline in your car, you must put living food into your body. Could this possibly be too difficult a concept to grasp?

In keeping with my promise to keep things simple and unencumbered, I am going to simplify another area that seems to confuse those people who want to know how much of what food group should be eaten so as to help them lose weight. High protein, low protein, all protein, no protein. High carb, low carb, no carbs. Fruits, fats, sugar. No matter how much of each a program, person or book recommends we consume, someone somewhere says just the opposite. I can see why people want to tear their hair out from frustration.

In 1923, there were twelve food groups. Can you imagine? In 1941, it was reduced to seven food groups, and by 1960, the now famous (or infamous) four food groups became the standard. Even though four is far easier to deal with than twelve, it still has people confused. Let's clear it up right now. There are only two food groups you have to concern yourself with, not four. And you know what they are, don't you? Living food and dead food. Whichever you wish to be (living or dead), all you have to do is see to it that your diet is predominated by foods from that group. What could be easier?

With the passage of time, as you become more familiar with the concept of eating more living food than dead food, or shall we say, cooked food (as they are synonymous), it will become increasingly clear to you what a freeing way of life it is. Eating not only remains a joy, as you are not "prohibited" from eating *any* food, but simultaneously it also brings your body to a healthy weight. Now, when I state that no foods are forbidden that is not to imply, as some temporary, ill-conceived diets sometimes suggest, that you can "eat all the steak, pizza and cheesecake you want and still lose weight." Not that you can't eat steak, pizza and cheesecake if you want; you *can*, but what you will come to learn is that it is the *amount* of these foods you eat compared to the amount of living food you eat that matters. It is the balance between these two foods, living and cooked, that is crucial.

Of course, the question most on your mind has to be, "Well, for optimum results, what *is* the ideal balance?" That is, indeed, the most important question, and I will answer it in the next chapter along with the other particulars that will help you reach the goal of predominating your diet with living food so as to normalize your weight and improve your overall well-being.

I think it is a trait of human nature to want proof when presented with new concepts, ideas and theories that challenge prevailing thought. In the area of health, well-being, weight loss and the like, that is invariably the case. Owing to the long line of disappointments people have endured with all manner of weight-loss schemes that have come and gone, it is completely understandable that people would want some proof that this approach will work. You're probably wondering, "Where's the science?"

That the premise presented is physiologically sound, there can be no doubt. You do not have to be a scientist to grasp the wisdom of providing the living body with living food. And although the greatest proof of all is in the doing, thereby *seeing* firsthand if it works for yourself, I do have a couple of offerings that will lend credence to the guiding principle that is being recommended.

The first is of a scientific nature. Before sharing it, I want to state clearly that, although I do rely on scientific studies to substantiate some of my work, I don't consider science to be the end-all and be-all. After all, science declares that there is no proof that there's a God. History is rife with examples of science declaring something to be or not to be so, only to find out later that it was wrong. It was once scientific dogma that the sun circled the Earth and not the other way around. Science once declared that smoking was a harmless habit, even recommended it for better digestion. Most everyone has heard of the scientific study that determined that a bumblebee's wings are not strong enough to carry its weight and therefore can't fly. Someone forgot to tell the bumblebee, however.

Mere unorthodoxy or dissent
from the prevailing mores is not to be
condemned. The absence of such voices
would be a symptom of grave
illness in our society.

—EARL WARREN

I have known scientists to reject out-of-hand theories that were not proven by double-blind studies. Yet they employ chemotherapy, which has never had a single double-blind study proving its worth. The all-time example of the value of scientific studies being suspect, if not outright worthless, appeared in the *New England Journal of Medicine*,[2] easily considered to be one of the most respected and prestigious scientific journals in the world. Two studies appeared in the very same journal, preceded by an apology from the editor. Both studies were impeccably conducted and therefore merited publication. The only thing was the two studies, although apparently sound, contradicted one another entirely. The two studies had to do with the use of hormones prescribed to postmenopausal women. One study "proved" that hormone therapy dramatically *increased* heart attacks; the other "proved" that it dramatically *decreased* heart attacks.

It is not my intention to imply that all scientific studies are to be regarded with suspicion; it would be foolish not to acknowledge that most are sound and useful. Sometimes studies come along that are so impressive in every way that they are hailed by one and all. And it is one of these that I wish to share with you here. Although this study has one of those protracted titles, over time it has come to be known as "Pottenger's Cats."[3] I would not be surprised if you have heard of this study in the past as it has been referred to in bibliographies in many health books. I have referred to it in at least two of my previous books.

Dr. Francis Pottenger conducted a meticulous, long-running experiment for the purpose of determining the effect of living food over cooked food. The reason I am so enamored of this study is because it is so uncomplicated and straightforward, with very few variables that could raise questions of its reliability.

Here's how it went: Over a period of at least ten years, Dr. Pottenger fed two groups of cats a diet that consisted of meat and milk and absolutely nothing else. One group was fed the meat and milk in a raw state, and the other group was fed the meat and milk cooked. That was it; no other variables came into play. It was meat and milk either raw or cooked and nothing else. The results were so overwhelmingly conclusive that there could be no doubt whatever of living food's superiority over cooked food. The cats fed only the living, uncooked food produced healthy offspring year after year. There was *no* ill health, disease or premature death, generation after generation. The cats fed the cooked food developed every one of humanity's modern ailments. The excrement from these cats was so toxic that weeds would not grow in the soil fertilized with it, whereas weeds proliferated in the stools from the cats fed the living, uncooked food. The first generation of kittens born to the cats that were fed only cooked food was sick and abnormal. The second generation was often born diseased or dead. By the third generation, the mothers were sterile. Dr. Pottenger conducted similar tests on mice, and the results coincided exactly with those of the tests run on cats.

The second piece of evidence I would like to offer to substantiate living food's superiority over cooked food is of a more esoteric nature. Like so many other people, I have long studied my spiritual side and contemplated my relationship with God and life, seeking answers to the age-old questions, "Who am I?" and "What am I doing here?" I have read the texts of numerous disciplines and religions and marvel at how similar they all are when it comes down to the basic question of how to live in a God-conscious way. Whether the Bible (Old or New Testament), the Bhagavad-Gita or the Koran, the message contained within all revolve around love, peace, mercy, kindness, forgiveness and nonjudgmental acceptance of one and all. I think if Jesus, Moses, Buddha, Lao-tzu, Mohammed and Confucius were all sitting around a table talking, they would find very little, if anything, to disagree upon. Reaching the top of the mountain is the goal; which path is taken is really secondary in importance to actually attaining the summit. In my desire to read as much on the subject as I could from as many different points of view as possible, I came across something I simply must share with you.

You are perhaps familiar with the Dead Sea Scrolls. They were found in the Judean desert along the shores of the Dead Sea in a place called Qumran in 1941. More than eight hundred manuscripts preserved for over two thousand years, the scrolls are some of the oldest biblical texts ever found. They were written by a sect known as the Essenes who lived during the time of Jesus and wrote manuscripts about him, his works and his words. In a small book entitled the *Essene Gospel of Peace*[4] are translations of conversations between Jesus and some of his followers. In one discourse, he was asked to discuss the manner in which food should be taken. As I was reading this, the following jumped off the page at me: "Kill (not) the food that goes into your mouth. For if you eat living food the same will quicken you, but if you kill your food the dead food will kill you also. For life comes only from life, and from death comes always death. For everything which kills your foods, kills your bodies also. . . . Therefore, eat not anything which fire has destroyed. . . . For your body is that which you eat." Wow! Considering the theme of this book, can you imagine the way my heart was racing when I read that?

If you have been grappling with your weight, then it is highly likely you have undertaken various weight-loss plans based on proof, testimonials, etc. The truth is, the proof I give, or any other type of proof based on statistics and the experience of others, can only tell you of the *potential* good that can be expected. There are no guarantees. Any given program may work well for one person but not for another. And that is because there are so many variables that come into play with each individual. The best proof there is, the most reliable proof, is results. You need to put the principle into practice and see for yourself if it's right for you.

I do not feel obliged to believe
that the same God who has endowed us
with sense, reason and intellect has
intended us to forgo their use.

—GALILEO

We have all been blessed at birth with common sense, and it is one of our greatest allies. Even though what you read here may be different and may appear to be overly simplistic, if it at least makes sense to you on the surface, if it does not assault your sense of logic and reason, that is a gigantic first step. I can't guarantee that you will be successful if you give it a try, and it would be misleading of me to do so. But I *can* assure you of one thing. I have been assisting people in losing weight and improving their health with the eating of more living food than cooked food for nearly thirty-five years, and I can't count the number of successes, including my own. All I can hope for is that you will be sufficiently intrigued enough to give it a fair trial.

I will tell you that there has been a colossal blunder in the long quest to conquer the problem of overweight, and mark my words it will go down as one of the most astonishing oversights in the history of the health sciences. I am talking about the failure to recognize and utilize the dynamics and intelligence of the living body.

The living body is powerful and capable beyond our comprehension. There isn't a scientist alive who is not in awe of the incomparable intelligence that governs all the activities of the living body. There isn't a scientist alive who can fully explain how the living body does what it does. The process of turning food into blood, bone, skin, muscle, teeth, hair and organs is itself such an extraordinary feat that it humbles all who are involved in the study of the living sciences.

The study of the human brain has been compared to studying the cosmos. As much as *is* known of this remarkable organ, we are still in the embryonic stages of understanding its magnificence. It is said that, with all we have accomplished on this planet, we use only 10 percent of our brain's potential. Some estimates say we use only 1 percent. So what is the other 90 percent of our amazing brain doing? The living body's natural, instinctive, inborn desire is for self-preservation. It can't help but strive for the highest level of well-being possible. It is incumbent upon anyone who desires to lose weight to learn how to unleash this untapped resource that resides inside the living body and allow it to do what it can do better than any diet, device or drug could ever hope to achieve.

We must learn how to get out of the body's way and allow it to attain the well-being it *automatically* strives for. We do this by fueling the body properly so it can do its work. The fuel is, of course, living food. And as you begin to change the balance of your food intake so that more living food is eaten than cooked food, you will have the great good fortune of seeing your body go to work at *optimum* efficiency, perhaps for the first time in your life. And then, look out! You are in for a very pleasant surprise.

Can you imagine what it would be like trying to describe the fragrant perfume of a rose to someone who had never actually smelled one? Even the most beautifully descriptive words possible would not come close to what actually smelling the rose would accomplish.

Until you experience firsthand the results of predominating your diet with living food, any description I give you, any attempt I make to have you grasp the good that can be expected, is doomed to fall short. It would be like trying to describe the scent of a rose to you without you ever having experienced it for yourself.

I spoke earlier of not expecting to find within these pages unrealistic promises of results that fly in the face of reason. No magic, no miracles. The true miracle is your living body and what it is capable of, given the opportunity to operate at its highest level, unencumbered of the burden of being forced to function on a diet predominated by dead food. Anyone can experience what are seemingly miraculous results by honoring his or her remarkable living body with a diet predominated by living food. Millions of people have found this out for themselves. On numerous occasions over the years, people have told me specifically that the introduction of more living food into their eating lifestyle has been a miracle in their lives. It is my sincerest wish that you will join their ranks.

CHAPTER THREE

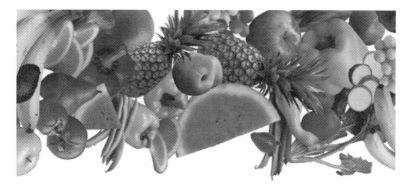

INTRODUCTION TO
THE KEYS TO SUCCESS

That which seems the height
of absurdity in one generation often
becomes the height of wisdom
in another.

—ADLAI STEVENSON

What a wonderful and exhilarating feeling it is to come upon some new piece of information with which you immediately resonate and see the possibilities of improvement it can bring into your life. Certainly, there must be those among you who, upon grasping the extreme importance of eating more living food than cooked food, which was imparted in the last chapter, must be excited at the prospect of something so apparently simple having the potential to accomplish so much.

I know it was like that for me in 1970 when I was first introduced to the concept of predominating my diet with living food. The timing could not have been better. To merely say I was desperate is a gross understatement. My father had died of cancer of the stomach after complaining of violent stomach pains for years. I also had violent stomach pains that required medication and kept me doubled over from the time I was three until I was twenty-five. I suffered from migraine headaches, I had no energy, and I was fifty pounds overweight after years of dieting.

The person who first told me about the need for living food did with me exactly what I told you I did with the people who ultimately came to me for help: He had me list everything in my diet no matter how much or how little I ate. What a shocker! It turned out I was *below* the average of 10 percent living food. No wonder I felt barely alive.

Thank heavens I have always loved fruit, which I considered to be a treat. So every so often I would have some. Salad, which I rarely ate as it would take up valuable stomach space that I would rather fill with a corn dog and onion rings, was a wedge of iceberg lettuce with a glob of mayonnaise. Days, literally, *days*, would go by when I would eat *nothing* living except for the slice of tomato on my cheeseburger. I remember the look on his face as he was reading over my list. It wasn't condescending, but he was slowly, almost imperceptibly, moving his head back and forth as he pursed his lips and rubbed his chin with his hand. Then he looked up at me with this look that I'll remember for all my days. "What?" I asked. "Why are you looking at me like that?" Not only had he seen it all before, but he was also marveling at the fact that there wasn't even more wrong with me considering the lifeless diet I was trying to exist on. It was as though he was getting ready to give me last rites.

Then he shared with me the contents of the previous chapter, and my life was forever changed. The proverbial lightbulb went off over my head—a lightbulb the size of a hot-air balloon. Even as I am writing about it now, that same surge of initial excitement I felt then is filling my body. I was obviously destined to learn this information because I wasn't the least bit skeptical of what he told me. I had no doubts or misgivings whatsoever about the credibility of what he was telling me. I simply felt that God had answered my prayers. Not a moment was wasted putting the principles into practice.

One month later I was unrecognizable from my former self. My skin, which was pallid before, glowed. My eyes sparkled. I stopped having headaches. The stomach ailment that plagued me my entire life was gone, and my energy level was "through the roof." And I was fifty pounds lighter! My entire outlook changed. I felt alive.

Now, I don't want to imply that all I had to do was *hear* what the solutions to my woes were and it all just magically changed. It would not be overstating it in the least to say that my motivation for change could not possibly have been greater. Remember, I was sick, in pain, tired, overweight, frustrated, and my father had died after exhibiting the very same symptoms I was experiencing. I could not have been more disgusted or disappointed with the string of diets I had been on, one of which consisted of nothing but cottage cheese and celery. Of course, I lost weight, but so what? As soon as I started eating again all the weight came back. And then some. You know what I'm talking about.

I'm telling you all this because I want you to know that it's all well and good to accept the worthiness of something intellectually, but it's something else entirely to put it into practice, especially when it's something that is contrary to what you have been doing for years, or perhaps your entire life. Your success in altering your eating lifestyle so as to lose weight and keep it off for the rest of your life is going to depend on your level of desire and commitment.

Some people, perhaps you even know some of those to whom I'm referring, are addicted to cigarettes or alcohol. They genuinely and sincerely *want* to break the addiction and free themselves from the grasp of something that has a hold over them. In other words, *intellectually* they have acknowledged and accepted the wisdom and value of not smoking or drinking. They absolutely know that their lives will be better, healthier and happier and want to stop. But they're addicted and can't. A Herculean effort must be put forth with a Twelve-Step program or some other type of assistance, and even though commitment and desire are at their height, some people fail to be successful.

There is no love sincerer than
the love of food.

—GEORGE BERNARD SHAW

Here's a news flash hot off the presses: Cooked food can be every bit as addictive as cigarettes, alcohol or any other substance or activity. The difference is that we can live perfectly well without cigarettes and alcohol. We require food to stay alive. That people become addicted to cooked food isn't speculation, and it's not something I'm fabricating just to make a point. Hey, I could write a book on the subject. (Oh, that's right, I *am* writing a book on the subject.) There are millions of people addicted—hooked on cooked food—and they don't even know it. It's not as though I'm talking about something about which I know nothing. I know about it all too well. There is not a day of my life as far back as I can remember, right up to and including today, that I have not been addicted to cooked food. And it's highly likely some of you reading this right now are chiming in with, "You and me both, brother!" There was a time in my life when I would never, *ever* admit such a thing even to myself! "Me? The *Fit for Life* guy, addicted to food?" Now I'm writing it in a book so millions of people can read about it. It was just my ego that wouldn't allow me to acknowledge it before. But it's nothing to be ashamed about, as I once thought. I'm not alone in this. I'll bet there are more people who are addicted to cooked food than who aren't.

The plain fact is, everything is set up to addict us to cooked food. I look back on my own past to see how I became so hooked on cooked food and so indifferent toward living food, and it seems so obvious to me now. On the one hand I was completely ignorant of the most basic and fundamental needs of the living body. On the other was the incessant advertising of cooked food, no matter where I looked. And it is the same thing today, isn't it?

Turn on the television and what's advertised there? Fruit and vegetables—the living foods? Hardly. It's invariably a cooked or processed food. Hamburgers, pizza, grilled shrimp, cookies, candy, cereal, frozen meals—everything cooked. Again, not that I want to imply that you can't eat those foods—you can. But what about the foods that actually keep you alive and supply the body with what it needs to carry out all the vital functions of life? Where are the ads for them? Or even a *discussion* of them? When have you ever seen an ad to eat fruit? The closest thing is an ad to drink orange juice. And it is invariably talking about pasteurized juice. Pasteurization is a process of heating that is so intense that nothing alive could possibly survive, let alone the delicate enzymes that are the constituents of life. Ever seen an ad for eating salad? The only time a salad is shown in an ad is in the context of advertising some overprocessed salad dressing. Walk into an average grocery store and what do you see? You see thirty aisles of cooked, processed (thereby dead) food and a produce section shoved over on the side with the only living food in the entire store.

The rest of the world lives to eat,
while I eat to live.

—SOCRATES

It's all backwards. It's life we want. It's health we want. Yet we are constantly pushed and prodded, tempted and teased, seduced with every enticement imaginable to stuff ourselves on all the foods that satisfy only our taste buds and *nothing* that satisfies the needs of the living body. Walk down any street in the country and look around. Look at the shape of most people's bodies. More people are overweight than not. Six out of every ten adults are overweight. And I've already mentioned that more children are overweight today than any other time in history.

We Americans lead the world in what are referred to as the diseases of affluence. Those are heart disease, cancer, diabetes, osteoporosis and, of course, obesity. Ever hear this old saying? "If we're not careful, we're going to wind up where we're heading." In order to *not* wind up where we're heading, it is incumbent upon you as an individual to recognize that a significant change is necessary to alter the present direction.

I hope that what I'm about to say does not come across as condescending or patronizing. It's something that a lot of people say in many different circumstances so it tends to lose its impact because of its frequent use. As it happens, in this instance, it is too apropos to *not* use. It is this: If I can do this, anyone can.

I grew up thinking that "good" food was any food that I could get into my mouth and down my throat. To this day I obsess over food. I think about it all the time. I think about it at night when I go to bed and in the morning when I wake up. I think about my next meal in the middle of meals I'm eating. I have to be ever diligent with my diet or my weight will skyrocket. I shudder to think of what my weight would be were I not aware of the principles regarding living food and cooked food. And I thank God in heaven that I learned them and am able to enjoy completely all of the foods I love to eat and am still able to control my weight. What a blessing it is to learn that the ultimate solution to losing weight allows for the eating of all foods that I have grown accustomed to over the years, and I am not forced to go without any of them.

You can do the same thing. I am telling you that if I, who have been hooked on food all my life and waddled around with an extra fifty pounds because of it, can eat the foods that I love and still lose weight and keep it off, *you can, too!* And instead of it requiring you to suffer and throw you into turmoil by being forced to comply to a regimen that is based on deprivation and robs the eating experience of its joy, there is but one simple principle to serve as your guiding light: Provide your body with more living food than dead (cooked/processed) food.

All health practitioners the world over, regardless of their specific area of expertise, have as their primary objective the goal of achieving homeostasis, or balance, in their patients. Proper balance is the key in all endeavors of life. When all the systems and mechanisms of the body are in balance, that is when we can rightly expect them to function at optimum efficiency, thereby producing the highest level of health possible. And the proper balance of living food over cooked food is, as expressed in the previous chapter, of paramount importance to your success in not only losing weight, but also keeping it off.

So what is the proper balance? Obviously, from what you have read thus far, the goal is to eat more living food than cooked food. But how *much* more is the question.

Because this is, in all probability, a brand-new concept for you, it is altogether likely that you want to have an exact formula with the precise percentage of living food and cooked food delineated. That expectation comes from years of measuring portions, counting calories and other calculations to which you had to strictly adhere. It's not like that with this. I've told you all along that this is different. It is far more freeing and easygoing, which is exactly how it *should* be. It's not as though I'm not going to suggest specific percentages for you to strive for—I am. But first and foremost, it is absolutely crucial that you start—*now*—to cultivate the mind-set that this is a relaxed lifestyle adjustment that merely requires a certain amount of relearning that is achieved over time with *no* pressure or rigid guidelines that must be adhered to. In that regard, two points are so extremely important that they cannot possibly be overemphasized. Truly. I wish there was some specific words that I could use, or some way to have these two points highlighted in red with blinking lights around them, so as to impress upon you the supremely significant role they will play in your overall, long-term success.

The distance is nothing; it is only
the first step that is difficult.

—Mme. DuDeffand

---

1. **There is no rush.** THERE–IS–NO–RUSH. You have the rest of your life. You have been eating in a certain way for years—decades—your entire life. It's not something you're going to turn around in a month or two. Nor should you. There is a transition period that is necessary. Try to turn it around too quickly and you may find yourself frustrated and ready to give up altogether.

   There seems to be a quick-fix, I-want-it-right-now attitude in all things these days. There is not a time, day or night, when you can't turn on the television and see an infomercial hawking the latest fad "breakthrough" for shedding weight. All too frequently the people who are the architects of the latest wonder cure are on screen flailing their arms, veins standing out on the sides of their necks and talking with such unbridled enthusiasm you'd think they were hopped up on caffeine and speed, all designed to excite you to the point of near delirium over the discovery that this is truly the one!

The ads are peppered with testimonials from happy, satisfied customers explaining that, "The weight came off so fast I could hardly believe it," and "The pounds just melted away before my eyes," and "I've tried them all, but this one really works." And, of course, there are the obligatory before and after pictures. What you never see, however, are the *after* after pictures. The ones that show how all the weight came back in 95 percent of the cases. That's right: When there is dramatic, rapid weight loss achieved with drugs, meal replacements or deprivation, the weight, and then some, is put back on 95 percent of the time.

What would you prefer? To lose thirty pounds in a month and in six months be right back to where you started, not only with the weight back on, but also in need of yet another scheme by which you could take the weight back off? Or would you prefer to lose thirty pounds over a period of six months and have a lifelong plan for keeping it off? Because if you pay heed to what I am putting forth in this book and lose a mere five pounds a month, that's exactly where you'll be in six months: thirty pounds lighter and equipped with the information and experience to keep it off.

Which would you prefer: to make $3 million in a month and be broke in six months, or to take six months to make $3 million and set it up to provide you with income for life?

The key here is that speed is nothing—direction is everything. For decades the allure has been how quickly weight could be dropped with no regard whatsoever for the long-term integrity of the living body. Whether the weight loss increased or decreased your overall health, whether the weight loss stayed off or was put back on faster than the time it took to lose it, was not even in the equation. The only consideration has been how much and how fast. Where has that mentality gotten you? It's time now to do it right.

Intemperate eating kills more people than tobacco and alcohol, because it is the most widespread fault. If people knew how to eat properly they would retain their youthful resiliency much longer.

—HENRY FORD

As strange as it may sound, the fact is, we never learned how to eat. Obviously, I don't mean we never learned how to get food into our bodies—all indications are that we have learned how to do that all too well. What I mean is that for some peculiar reason, we never learned how to eat in a way that honored the living body and provided it with what it needed to function properly and exist in a harmonious state. To aspire to correct this blunder and make it right is a most noble endeavor and will be met with complete success—if you allow the change to unfold in a relaxed, unpressured manner without trying to remedy in too short a time a situation that took years to create.

2. **Results will be noticeable.** Having spent the last few paragraphs extolling the virtue of patience while rethinking and redefining the type of food that makes up your diet, and not trying to rush the process of re-directing it, I can understand if you might be saying, "Hey, that's fine, but frankly I need to drop some pounds *now!* And didn't you, only a few pages ago, say you lost fifty pounds in a month?" Yes, I did. But I want to assure you that my primary goal at the time was not weight loss. Oh, I wanted to lose weight *desperately*, but what I wanted even more desperately was to feel better. I was sick and in pain most of the time, and I'm going to share with you now what the person who first intro-duced me to the importance of eating more living food than cooked food told me then.

Being in pain, not having enough energy, being overweight, feeling poorly most of the time—these are all *symptoms* of a singular condition, that condition being a general state of ill health brought on by with-holding from the living body the proper fuel it needs (living food) to function properly. You can't be healthy and overweight at the same time. Oh, sure, I've heard people describe someone by saying, "You know, except for all that extra weight he/she's carrying around, he/she's really healthy." Wrong! You can no more be healthy and overweight than you can be wet and dry at the same time.

Those who have health have hope;
and those who have hope
have everything.

—ARABIAN PROVERB

As much as you want to lose weight, when you focus your attention on improving your body's overall health, that is when success with weight loss will come. The living body cannot help but to strive for its own highest state of well-being and self-preservation. It does so automatically as part of the life process. Health is natural; ill health is unnatural. The secret to losing weight, and this is something that you should never lose sight of, is that the living body does not have to be prompted to attain a level of health that precludes being overweight; it only needs to be given the *opportunity* to do so.

So here is the second monumentally important point I want to make that has to do with the results you so fervently desire. Even though the time necessary to fully retrain yourself to eating the way I am suggesting may take six months or a year or even longer, the *moment* you start to simultaneously increase the amount of living food and decrease the amount of cooked food, the living body immediately seizes upon that opportunity and starts to correct any imbalances that exist. And it is a sight to behold, as you shall see. When restraints are removed and the powerful, incomparable forces that govern the living body and all its activities are unleashed, results are assured.

Let's just say, for the sake of this discussion, that you are one of those who have been eating the norm of about 10 percent living food. So you're at 10 percent versus 90 percent (10 percent living food, 90 percent cooked food). Let's suppose your ultimate goal, two or three years down the road, is to be at 75 percent–25 percent, or 60 percent–40 percent, or whatever your goal happens to be. Your body will start making improvements the moment more living food is introduced with a similar reduction of cooked food. What that means is you could *double* the amount of living food you are presently eating to 20 percent–80 percent, and even though that may be a long way from your ultimate goal, twice the amount of living food your body is accustomed to is enough to ignite the body's healing mechanism in charge of producing the improved health and weight loss you desire.

I wish to share with you something enormously encouraging that you would understandably not be familiar with if over your lifetime your living food has been around the norm of 10 percent. It has to do with the rapidity with which the living body starts to correct all imbalances (including weight loss) at its first opportunity. It was only a few paragraphs ago that I made the point that the body doesn't have to be *forced* to fix itself. It's something the body does for its own self-preservation, automatically. To say that it is opportunistic is an understatement. The *moment* a doorway of opportunity is opened, the healing mechanism of the living body rushes headlong through it.

What I am talking about can be likened to the nature of water. When water is being contained by a dam, or behind a dike, or in a jar or an irrigation channel, the very instant an opening occurs, a crack or break or fissure of any kind, water instantaneously, very nearly *simultaneously*, enters that opening. There is not the slightest hesitation; it is immediate. And so it is with the living body, ever on alert to make whatever corrections are necessary in order to effect a positive change in its well-being.

This is not something that happens some of the time to only some of the people who establish these openings. It happens *all* the time and to *all* who create the environment within the body, such as when more living food is suddenly introduced into the diet. Perhaps you are thinking this is too bold a statement to make in light of the fact that not all strategies work for all people. I'm sure you are aware of those commercials that I referred to earlier, which are drenched with before and afters, testimonials and extravagant weight-loss successes that exclaim, "It is so effortless." They sound so fantastic that you give them a try only to find out that your results are nothing like the ones advertised. Why? It's a classic use of a partial truth that hooks you, but it's the full truth that ushers you back to reality. If you were to put a hundred people at random on one of these "miracle diets," what you would find is that perhaps 10 to 15 percent, at best, would do incredibly well even with moderate effort. On the other end of the spectrum, about 10 to 15 percent would do horribly, even with supreme effort and discipline. And about 70 percent would have varying levels of results. So about 15 percent have the kind of results advertised in the commercial, and about 85 percent are being set up for disappointment. That's because there are far too many variables that come into play to make the claims that are made. Individual metabolism, genetic makeup, physical activity and others, known and unknown, all come together to be the determining factor as to whether or not there will be success. Guess which 15 percent you see on the commercials?

There are, however, certain results that *always* happen, *all* the time to *all* people. If you cut yourself with a knife, you will bleed. If you swallow food, your digestive system will fire up and go to work digesting the food. If you don't take fluids into your body, you will become dehydrated. If you put your hand on a hot stove, it will burn. And if you double the amount of living food in your diet while simultaneously lowering your intake of cooked food, your living body, always seeking a way to acquire and maintain the highest level of health possible, *will* immediately initiate the cleansing and healing that is necessary in order to normalize your weight. And it will do this as quickly and efficiently as water flows into an opening. Remember, you cannot be healthy *and* overweight. And since the living body is always naturally and instinctively seeking to achieve good health, it must, of necessity, shed the weight that stands in its way.

So, here we are. What should your goal be? What is the ideal ratio of living food to cooked food that will allow you to enjoy the eating experience and not feel deprived or on a "diet," while simultaneously providing your body with the proper fuel it needs to shed your excess weight and maintain a consistent, high level of good health? Once again, that which is sensible, reasonable and practical rules the day. It's not as though I would ask you to reverse the percentages from 10 percent living food and 90 percent cooked food to 90 percent living food and 10 percent cooked food. Or for that matter, to strive for 80 percent to 20 percent or even 70 percent to 30 percent. No. Taking into account that the living body requires living food and the entire premise of this book is that one should therefore eat more living food, what could be more logical, realistic and reasonable than to suggest that it be half and half?

CHAPTER FOUR

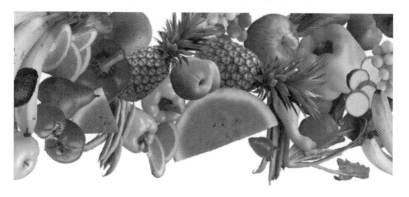

KEY TO SUCCESS #1:
50 PERCENT LIVING FOOD–
50 PERCENT COOKED FOOD

Our life is frittered away by detail.
Simplicity, simplicity,
simplicity!

—HENRY DAVID THOREAU

Please allow me to be brutally honest with you here; no pussyfooting around or tiptoeing around the subject so as not to offend. In no way do I want to offend, but I do want to be real. Considering that your success in losing weight and recapturing your health depends upon the amount of living food in your diet, if you are not willing to eat *at least* as much living food as you are willing to eat dead food, then you're not really serious about this. If you *are* serious and you set your sights on reaching the goal of one half your food intake being living, you're home free. By that I mean you get to do one of the things I know you want very much to do: *You get to eat!* No starvation, no drugs, no diets, no meal replacements, no special devices, no brutal workouts, no deprivation, no calorie-counting, no portion-measuring, no wondering about high protein/low protein or high carb/low carb—the entire list of tortures that customarily accompanies diets becomes completely irrelevant. How great is *that?* The one and *only* issue to be considered is, are you eating as much living food as you are cooked food? Short of kicking a magic lantern that releases a genie that grants you the wish of being just the weight you want to be, I can't think of anything simpler. Can you? Plus, and this is a great big, gigantic whopper of a plus, the other benefits you will enjoy, aside from weight loss, are numerous. You'll learn those in a later chapter. At the mere prospect that what I'm telling you does indeed work, and I have decades of experience *watching* it work in huge numbers of people's lives, you have reason to be celebrating your coming liberation right now.

Remember, just because you have intellectually accepted the wisdom of balancing the amount of living food to cooked food that you eat doesn't mean that you have to be at 50 percent–50 percent tomorrow. Not that I want to discourage you from going straight to 50 percent–50 percent. It would be fantastic, beyond fantastic, if you did. But the plain fact is, some people can make such abrupt alterations in their lifestyle with ease, while others require a transition period. Either way is fine. Don't forget, there is no rush. You have all the time you need, and noticeable, positive results will be apparent shortly after you start to increase your intake of living food while decreasing your intake of cooked food. This is especially so for those people who are even below the norm of 10 percent living food to 90 percent cooked food. I'm talking about those folks who eat less than 5 percent living food (i.e., everything else, over 95 percent of their diet, is cooked). These are the people who say, "I have a piece of fruit or a salad every other day or so." I weep for people who eat fruit and vegetables so infrequently. It is the cause of so much of their suffering, and they don't have a clue. But I'm encouraged by the fact that I know how much their lives are going to improve once they start to adopt the changes this book recommends. In fact, generally speaking, it is the people who eat the fewest fruits and vegetables who experience the most noticeable and rapid change as they start to supply the living food their bodies so desperately crave.

There is a question that I know is hovering in your mind at present because it is the same question asked by everyone introduced to this concept of 50 percent to 50 percent living food to cooked food. It goes something like this: "How do I know just how much living and cooked food I'm eating? What if I want to be at 50 percent but I'm only at 43.7 percent? How will I know?" The quick answer is, you won't. Not exactly and precisely, anyway. And that is part of the beauty and ease of this way of eating. As I have pointed out all along, this way of eating fits comfortably and conveniently into your life. In the past, I have personally found the measuring and calculating of portion sizes to be not only bothersome but also arduous and demeaning. It takes the fun right out of the eating experience. There is no need for you to ever think in terms of knowing the exact percentage of the food you are eating. This is one of those examples, like in horseshoes, where close *does* count.

Whenever I mention eating a certain percentage of food, either living or cooked, it is always an approximation. And that is all it needs to be for you to be successful. As far as you knowing when you've reached the desired mark you're seeking, *you'll know*. You're going to have to go on faith and trust me on this for now. After spending nearly three and a half decades teaching this concept to more people than I can recount, I can tell you there is a subtle transformation that takes place in people, and it *always* happens. As people become more and more familiar with the enormously significant role living food plays in all areas of their well-being, there is a certain "knowing" that comes into play. I'm not trying to be evasive or vague, but until you start to *experience* what I'm talking about, it is extremely difficult for me to convey now what you will undoubtedly understand later. It's like the example I gave earlier of not being able to fully appreciate the fragrant scent of a rose only by a verbal description. It has to be smelled—experienced—to be appreciated. It's the same thing here.

Do you remember ever getting a new computer, fax machine or VCR and being initially bewildered at the apparent complexity of its operation? Then after you used it for awhile, it became like second nature. You might even have commented, after becoming completely familiar with it, that, "This thing is so easy to use, I can't believe I ever thought it was confusing at first." Bingo! It's the same deal.

I already know that for those who introduce more living food into their diets (and decrease cooked food), successful results are realized. There's just no doubt about that. As to what degree of success these results will reach, only time will tell. There is no blanket declaration that can honestly be made. As stated earlier, different variables come into play for different people, and those are the determining factors. But I will tell you what the single most important ingredient is in achieving the results you desire: willingness. You need a willingness to make a commitment to change and follow through on that commitment—at least temporarily, until a determination of its worthiness can be made. You must be willing to cast aside every preconceived notion you may have about what should or should not be done dietetically to lose weight. Those who throw themselves with complete abandon and faith into this new approach to nourishing the body, having cut loose from all past concepts, will be the ones who enjoy the greatest rewards.

Action may not always bring happiness;
but there is no happiness
without action.

—Benjamin Disraeli

All you have to do is *start* and not worry about anything else. Don't get hung up on the percentages and exact amounts and measurements. Everything will fall into place and take care of itself once you have started putting into practice all that you have been given throughout the course of this book. Think of what it's like when you're watching a mystery movie that has a convoluted plot with twists and turns that keep you in the dark until the very end. Finally, when all the pieces have been put together, your confusion turns to order. In fact, in hindsight, you may even wonder why you weren't able to figure it all out sooner because it was all so obvious. It's something like that here. It may be confusing at first, but that's only because it's new and you don't know the end yet. After you have lived it for awhile, it will become second nature to you. Once again, all you have to do is start, and all your questions will be answered.

As I am relating all this to you, I can't help but reflect back to 1970, which was the first time I had ever heard of the idea of actually supplying the living body with the living food it needed to survive. At first, I was wondering how in the world I, a confirmed, inveterate cooked-food "junkie," was ever going to be able to go from about 5 percent living food and 95 percent cooked food to 50 percent living food and 50 percent cooked food. But because of the promise of ending all the pain I was living with, *plus* the prospect of losing the weight I had been wrestling with for years, I took the advice that was given to me then, which I am giving to you now. I trusted that it would all come together for me if I would just start. In terms of my health and well-being, following that advice was the wisest decision I ever made.

Even though my long-term goal was ultimately twice as much living food as cooked food, or about two-thirds living and one-third cooked, my immediate desire was to reach the goal of 50 percent–50 percent. Since I was expecting a lot from my body, I figured the very *least* I could do was support its efforts the best I could, and that meant giving it an ample amount of the proper fuel it needed to do what had to be done.

That day in 1970, I made a commitment to God and the universe that I would, from that day forward, see to it that at least half of my food intake was made up of living food. And because I have followed through on that commitment, I have reaped the rewards. For over thirty years, I have been able to eat the foods I like while maintaining a comfortable, manageable body weight.

Interestingly, I happen to have the perfect body type for testing this way of eating. My body is extremely responsive to changes in my diet. This actually has been a blessing and a curse for me. I can put on four pounds by reading a menu. This is obviously an exaggeration, but my point is that the slightest dietary indiscretions cause me to gain weight, but I lose that weight rapidly by doing what I know is right. So over the years, whenever I would, for whatever reason, start to eat less living food than cooked food, sure enough, the weight would creep back on. And as soon as I would go back to 50 percent (or more) living food, the weight would fall right back off. I can scarcely relate how liberating and exhilarating it is to know that it's not some external influence out of my control that is in charge of whether or not I am overweight. *I* am in charge. *I* am the one in control. I wish this feeling for you, and if you will utilize the keys to success I am presenting, you can happily find out firsthand exactly what I'm talking about.

There is no failure except
in no longer trying.

—KIN HUBBARD

CHAPTER FIVE

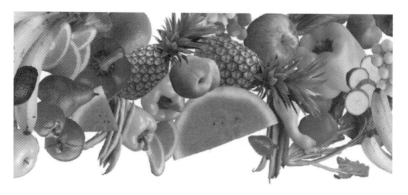

KEY TO SUCCESS #2:
BE FRUITFUL AND FLOURISH

Whenever a new discovery is
reported to the scientific world, they say first,
"It is probably not true." Thereafter, when the
truth of the new proposition has been
demonstrated beyond question, they say,
"Yes, it may be true, but it is not important."
Finally, when sufficient time has elapsed to
fully evidence its importance, they say,
"Yes, surely it is important,
but it is not new."

—CHARLES AUGUSTIN MONTAIGNE

Over the years I have given hundreds of interviews—perhaps more than a thousand including television, radio and print. I've been asked every question imaginable and some you would never imagine. There are two questions in particular I have been asked with such regularity that you might think they were required to be asked. Certainly they have been asked more often than any other. They are: (1) "What is the single most important dietary principle you have ever learned in your years of study?" and (2) "What are the absolute best and absolute worst foods you can put into your body?" I can think of no other questions that are easier to answer. They are as obvious as the answer to the question, "Where would you find more glaciers, on the equator or the Antarctic?"

A little later, we'll discuss what the worst food is, in my opinion, in the human diet. But for now, in order to reveal the second key to success, I want to discuss the food that is not only at the heart of the most important dietary principle I have ever learned, but is also the best and finest food you can possibly eat: fruit!

Whenever the subject of fruit is being talked about, two thoughts immediately come to mind for me. The first is Mark Twain's statement: "There are two things that are infinite: space and man's stupidity." The second is the mind-boggling ignorance exhibited about the true nature of fruit by those so-called "experts" or "authorities" who really ought to know better. There *is* no more perfect food available to us on this planet than fruit. Once you have learned about its unique nature and the guidelines that govern the correct way of eating it (yes, there is a correct and incorrect way to eat fruit), you will then be able to make use of this most supreme culinary gift from God to help achieve all of your health goals, including weight loss. Nothing I am saying, or will say, about how instrumental fruit will be in helping you achieve all your health goals is an exaggeration. If anything, no matter how highly I praise it, it will fall short of the true nature of this astonishing food.

One of the more exhilarating and wondrous aspects of life is when we are fortunate enough to discover some brand-new, previously unknown piece of information that obviously and dramatically improves our life in some way, whether in the arena of health, spiritual awareness, our love life, finances or relationships. It is most rewarding when that new information proves itself to have a verifiable, positive influence on the length and quality of life. For millions of people, myself included, the discovery of the principles that govern the proper consumption of fruit has been nothing short of a blessing of the highest order.

If you should take only *one* thing from this book, make it this. Truly, if you were to take to heart explicitly the recommendations made in this section on fruit, and you did absolutely *nothing* else, you would realize a definite and clearly noticeable improvement in all areas of your well-being.

> I am too much of a skeptic to deny
> the possibility of anything.
>
> —T. H. Huxley

If this assertion about fruit is brand-new to you, perhaps you are skeptical or at least interested in hearing the substantiating evidence that leads me to declare this with such certainty. And since I am placing such extreme importance on this one factor, I think it would be instructive to share with you, briefly, how I became so totally convinced of the health-promoting nature of fruit.

In 1970 when I first learned of the benefits of fruit and the extent to which it could help me lose weight and regain my health, I just jumped right in. I took seriously the admonition from my mentor not to digress one iota from the guidelines that dictate how fruit should and should not be eaten. He *promised* me that if I listened to what he shared with me concerning fruit, that I would not only lose weight and dramatically improve my health, but that I would ultimately one day acknowledge what I learned about fruit to be the greatest health discovery of my life. He said all of this with such conviction and enthusiasm that I felt like I would be committing treason if I didn't follow his advice. I assured him that whatever else I might do or not do in terms of the advice he was giving me on diet, as far as eating fruit, I would not deviate from the principles he suggested even to the slightest degree. I followed through on that promise, and the powerful, health-promoting benefits of eating fruit correctly quickly became obvious to me.

Over the next ten years (1970–1980) I continued following the dietary principles I learned, and I immersed myself in the study of Natural Hygiene, the field that encompasses these principles. Although on occasion I would waver with some of the principles of proper diet, not so with the ones governing the correct eating of fruit that I held to be sacred, for lack of a better term.

During this time, I not only shared this information with family and friends, I also started to counsel people one-on-one, always placing added emphasis on the importance of adhering most closely to the principles related to eating fruit correctly. This is when I started to get feedback from people that mirrored my own experience: Eating fruit properly brought results that were immediate and long-lasting.

It was becoming increasingly obvious to me that the correct consumption of fruit held enormous, health-enhancing possibilities that were virtually unknown to the vast majority of the population. Although this was glaringly obvious to me, it was based on the experience of only a couple of hundred people or so. Impressive, yes, but not nearly enough to "stop the presses" or shout it from the mountaintops.

Then in mid-1980, I had the extreme good fortune to meet and work with one of the most remarkable people I have ever known: Anthony Robbins. This was when Tony was only twenty-one and had not yet conquered the world. After familiarizing himself with my work and applying the dietary principles that obviously appealed to his common sense and brought an immediate improvement in his health, he decided to bring to bear his formidable talents and help bring this life-saving information to a larger audience. Since *Fit for Life* had not yet been written, his idea was that I should start to conduct public seminars that he would promote and administer. I quickly nixed that idea because I had a paralyzing fear of public speaking, having once thrown up on myself in oral-communications class in high school when forced to address the class. "That's great!"—so said Tony who, as you may or may not know, is probably the world's leading practitioner in helping people overcome their deepest fears. As far as he was concerned, my giving seminars would not only help get the good word out, but also allow me to conquer my fear of public speaking. It is virtually impossible to be in the presence of Tony's super-positive, there's-no-such-thing-as-can't attitude and not make positive changes in your life. The seminars, it turns out, were highly successful, and between my own genuine enthusiasm for the information and Tony's guidance, I turned out to be pretty good at it.

The block of granite, which is an obstacle in the pathway of the weak, becomes a stepping-stone in the pathway of the strong.

—THOMAS CARLYLE

After a few years of that, I had thousands of people giving me feedback on how the dietary changes I recommended were impacting their lives. Sure enough, the most frequent comment I heard revolved around the effects of eating fruit properly.

In June 1985, *Fit for Life* was published, and thanks to its straightforward, common-sense approach, word of its effectiveness quickly spread. The book skyrocketed to number one on the *New York Times* bestseller list, where it remained for an unprecedented forty straight weeks. It has racked up some 12 million sales and, to this day, nearly twenty years later, it still sells around 100,000 copies a year worldwide, in seventy countries and thirty-three languages.

I no longer had to depend on the feedback of a few hundred or even a few thousand people to validate my belief that eating fruit correctly held the potential to transform one's life. From 1985 until today, I have received some 600,000 communications from people commenting on and asking questions about *Fit for Life*. People continue to write, fax, e-mail, phone and stop me on the street to share their experiences with me. And wouldn't you know it, far and away the most frequent subject referred to has to do with fruit. In fact, there have been more comments about one aspect or another pertaining to the positive effects of eating fruit correctly than all other comments on all other subjects *combined!* Any little hint of doubt I may have been harboring that perhaps I was just projecting my own positiveness and desires onto the subject were obliterated. To have such a huge number of people, hundreds of thousands, from all walks of life, from all around the world, relate such similar experiences was more powerfully convincing than anything I could have possibly come up with on my own. To reiterate: Nothing in this book will do more to help you lose weight and optimize your health than following as closely as you can the suggestions on how and when to eat fruit correctly. If you will do so, you, too, can be happy for the remainder of your fit, trim and healthy life.

The three primary religions of India are Hinduism, Buddhism and Jainism. There are at present approximately 7 million Jains living to one degree or another by the 3,000-year-old tradition of Ahimsa, or nonviolence. Mahatma Gandhi was a proponent of Jainism. Jains, under no circumstances, do anything in any way to harm any living being, large or small. It is their religion to live in peace and harmony with all living things.

The more orthodox go so far as to wear masks over their mouths so as not to breathe in and kill tiny insects or organisms they can't see. As amazing as that is, there are those Jains, few in number to be sure, who are even *more* strict, if you can believe that. There are those who have taken the concept of nonviolence to the absolute extreme. They will kill nothing that's alive, including plants! This severely narrows down their food choices.

It goes without saying that no Jain would eat anything from the animal kingdom, so that leaves the plant kingdom. But whether it's lettuce or carrots or broccoli or onions or potatoes, all have to be taken from the plant before they have completed their growing process, or as a Jain would say, "Before God finished with it." If left alone, all would go to seed and flower.

There is one food, however, that God *does* "finish with." Once this food has grown to its absolute fullest potential and can grow no more, it either withers or dies on the tree or vine or falls from the tree or vine. Of course, I'm referring to fruit. There are Jains who literally do not eat on days in which no fruit has fallen from the trees they frequent. If I were one of those Jains, you would generally be able to find me up in a tree wildly shaking the branches like a crazed orangutan.

I honestly believe that it is
better to know nothing than to
know what ain't so.

—JOSH BILLINGS

As far as food for the human species is concerned, fruit is the most perfect, most beneficial, most health-promoting food on our planet. Anyone who would tell you differently—or would, worse yet, have you avoid fruit altogether, as is suggested in the all-protein death diets—is guilty of the most inexcusable ignorance of the physiological and biological needs of life.

A strong case could be made that the very first and most important line of defense that we humans have to protect ourselves against anything harmful entering our bodies is our senses. Is fruit not a veritable celebration for the senses? If something looks repulsive, would you be inclined to eat it? If something smells foul, would you be tempted to put it in your mouth? If something tastes nasty, would you chew it up and swallow it? Fruit is the exact antithesis of this. It is inviting in every way. Is there anything quite so aromatic and enticing as the sweet scent of a fully ripe peach? Can anything surpass the luscious flavor of a fresh-cut slice of watermelon on a hot day? And, of course, fruit is a feast for the eyes. Is there anywhere to be found an artist's palate that can rival the spectacular circus of colors that a table laden with a wide variety of fruit can display? As important as it is for fruit to pass the test of the senses with such high marks, it is only the hem of the garment—there is so very much more.

Because there is a seemingly endless number of different types and varieties of food to be eaten, I think we tend to lose sight of the primary purpose of eating. We are, first and foremost, living beings, and we must eat food in order to remain alive. That is why we must eat. *To live!* And in an act of pure genius the Grand Creator gifted us with taste buds to make the eating experience enticing and enjoyable, as well as life-giving. We can only imagine what food would be like if we didn't have taste buds—a nutrient-rich, cardboard-like mush that we would simply shove in as quickly as possible in order to be done with the task. It would all look the same and all be the same since it would have one purpose: to supply our bodies with the nutrients and the energy required to live. If that were the case, we sure wouldn't need books like this one. I would either be writing on a different subject or be doing stand-up at The Improv.

Let the stoics say what they please;
we do not eat for the good of living, but
because the food is savory and
the appetite is keen.

—Ralph Waldo Emerson

As glorious a gift as it is to have taste buds in order to enjoy fully the eating experience, those taste buds, without a doubt, have been a source of both pleasure and pain. Because there is what appears to be an infinite variety of tasty and delectable vittles to be had, the tendency has become all too common to eat for the sake of satisfying the taste buds while giving barely a second thought to what the body needs to survive. And, alas, I'm afraid that is the very reason why so many people find themselves struggling to lose weight.

Have you ever overheard or participated in a conversation such as this?

"I haven't eaten yet. Want to go to lunch?"

"Yes, I'm starving. Where do you want to go?"

"There's a place around the corner that has a menu full of items that nourishes the body with all the nutrients we need, plus it helps flush out built-up toxins from the system."

"Sounds great, let's do it."

Yeah, right. Now, I'm not suggesting that we eat only foods that nourish us and nothing that only pleases the taste buds. Nor am I suggesting that the foods that are most nourishing don't also tantalize the taste buds, because they do. But let's face it: The plain fact is, most people think *only* of what will taste good and rarely, if ever, make their food choices based on what the body needs to function well and survive. And that is why most people eat less than 10 percent living food and more than 90 percent cooked food.

Fruit tops the list when it comes to supplying the living body with everything it needs to carry out all the vital functions of life with the greatest ease, energy and efficiency. Notwithstanding the pleasure we receive from enjoying a delicious meal of savory and flavorful food, to stay alive and thrive healthfully, we must eat in order to obtain the two vital elements that perpetuate life: nutrients and energy.

All the vitamins, minerals, amino acids for protein, fatty acids, phytonutrients, antioxidants, in fact, every substance or compound known to support and promote life, are resplendent in fruit. And *if* eaten correctly, fruit will provide your body with everything it needs to live healthfully.

Energy and persistence
conquer all things.

—BENJAMIN FRANKLIN

The true test of the worthiness of any food is the energy value for the body, measured against the energy required for it to be digested and metabolized. And it is in this test that the true superiority and magnificence of fruit shines most brightly. We are, after all, living energy systems. Without energy, what would we be? We wouldn't be able to move, breathe, swallow, digest food, stand up or sit down, walk, talk, blink our eyes, *nothing!* Since the energy we need to fuel these activities, and literally millions more, is derived from the food we eat, we owe it to ourselves to eat those foods that are not only a source of energy, but are also the foods from which energy can be most efficiently extracted and utilized.

It is impossible to discuss the securement and use of energy without also discussing the most studied, yet least understood, complex and awe-inspiring organ of the human body: the brain. To even begin to comprehend the magnitude of the brain's mastery and the cooperativeness of each one of the approximately 100 trillion cells under its command, we would have to possess an intellect infinitely more developed than it is at present. This is why there are many scientists who have dedicated their lives to the study of the brain yet are firmly convinced that the true magnificence of this astonishing marvel of creation will never be fully understood.

> The brain is Nature's
> supreme achievement.
>
> —FRIEDRICH NIETZSCHE

In order to give you a mere inkling, a hint, of the incomprehensible ability of the brain and what it is capable of, consider this: In today's climate of strife and turmoil, imagine a thousand people from each country of the world getting together and cooperating harmoniously in all things. If that seems difficult then now imagine all 6.5 billion inhabitants of the Earth together acting and thinking in complete unison. Although such a possibility seems absurd, compared to the human body with all its cells, and the brain at its helm, that would be nothing! Try to picture 15,000 Earths each with 6.5 billion people all acting as one in total alignment with one another functioning as a single, unified whole. Only with such staggering thoughts as these is it possible to grasp some idea and have some sense of what the human brain is capable of achieving. For indeed, the brain manages to coordinate flawlessly the prodigious number of actions and activities of every last one of the 100 trillion cells so as to work in perfect harmony with one another.

No computer in existence could possibly perform the astronomical number of functions conducted by the brain. It oversees every last activity of the body: It manufactures blood as needed, and the heart pumps 100,000 times a day, sending six quarts of it through over 90,000 miles of blood vessels; every organ works with precision and in concert with every other organ; temperature is maintained; balance is maintained; food is digested; nutrients are extracted; wastes are removed; respiration supplies oxygen to every cell; all senses operate; the immune system, nervous system and musculoskeletal system all perform their duties; and more activities too numerous to name are all being carried out with pinpoint precision every moment, twenty-four hours a day for a hundred years or more if need be. It's mind-boggling!

It seems unnecessary to mention, in fact almost absurd to point out, that whatever fuel energy the brain requires to perform at optimum effectiveness should be supplied in its purest form, its most easily accessible form and in the form that can be most efficiently utilized. And what is the fuel required by the brain to produce the energy necessary to "stoke the engines," so to speak? In a word, sugar—namely, glucose. Anytime you see a word that ends in -ose (glucose, sucrose, fructose, etc.), it's a type of sugar. The type of sugar that the brain needs as fuel is glucose, and that is the one and *only* fuel the brain can use. It can't burn protein directly, it can't burn fats directly, and it can't burn starches directly. Whatever is taken into the body must ultimately be broken down into glucose before the brain can use it. The reason so many people have a "sweet tooth" is that it is our natural inclination. Obviously, the question of most importance is, what provides the brain with the finest source of glucose with the least expenditure of energy to obtain it?

There are three major components of living matter: protein, fats and carbohydrates. The primary use of protein in the body is to build, repair and maintain living tissue. The primary use of fat in the body is for heat, padding and insulation for organs and as regulator of the fat-soluble vitamins, A, D, E and K. The primary use of carbohydrates—no, check that—not the primary use, but the *only* use of carbohydrates in the body, is for fuel energy. There is not a single living thing, plant or animal, that does not contain carbohydrates in some form. Life as we know it could not exist without them. Carbohydrates are the principal source of energy for human beings. The human body has been designed and built by you-know-who to consume carbohydrates, in order to obtain the fuel energy it needs to conduct all the processes of life and without which all body functions would cease—death would occur. Right about here it would be so easy to get all bogged down in a long, drawn-out, convoluted and technical explanation of the multiple processes that take place to convert foods into glucose so the brain would have access to it. Pages could be written describing and defining all the different stages and the numerous, multisyllabic words you're probably not even familiar with that are used to describe all the activities involved in turning food into energy. Frankly, it's pretty boring stuff to read, so I'm not going to go there. Anyone interested in that aspect of the subject can certainly pick up a book on physiology and read all about it.

There is, however, one word with which I do have to familiarize you so you can fully grasp and understand the exceedingly important point I am making here about our body's need for carbohydrates. The word is saccharide (pronounced "sack-a-ride"). I promise to keep it short and simple. A saccharide is another way of saying carbohydrate. The three primary classifications of saccharides (carbohydrates) are monosaccharides, which contain one molecule of carbohydrate; disaccharides, which contain two molecules of carbohydrate; and polysaccharides, which contain three or more molecules of carbohydrate. The body (brain) can use only monosaccharides, the most simple, least complex of all carbohydrates. And until any food or substance in the body is broken down into its simplest form, a monosaccharide, it cannot and will not be available for use as fuel. There, that's all the technical stuff.

You've learned that the *only* fuel the brain can use to produce energy is a form of sugar called glucose. Glucose *is* a monosaccharide. All foods are a source of carbohydrates, but some are better than others, meaning the less effort and energy the body has to expend to turn something, anything, into glucose (a monosaccharide) the better. Protein and fat *can* be used, but *only* indirectly by first being converted into a carbohydrate and then into a monosaccharide. And this only takes place when carbohydrate intake is inadequate. You must never lose touch with the fact that the human body wants, needs and *must have* carbohydrates to survive. The infinite intelligence that governs all activities of the body is provident, which means it is always concerned with its self-preservation and has mechanisms in place to protect itself. It has many backup arrangements for survival in emergency situations when sufficient carbohydrates are not available. That is why there is a process in place that will convert proteins and fats into carbohydrates. But at what cost? The body only has a limited amount of energy available at any given time, and a considerable amount of it is used up in this conversion process. Energy that could have been used for other vital tasks such as cleansing and strengthening the body or losing weight is squandered unnecessarily.

There's a mighty big difference
between good, sound reasons and
reasons that sound good.

—BURTON HILLIS

This is why the all-protein diets are so dangerous. They are classic, textbook examples of "weight loss at any cost." They will result in weight loss, but it is with no regard for the damage that may be done to a person's health. Weight loss is achieved by so severely restricting carbohydrates that it tricks the body into thinking it's sick. Let me explain. If you look through the *Merck Manual*, which is an encyclopedia of the thousands of possible illnesses the human body can experience, you will notice that the one most common symptom of disease is the loss of appetite. The more catastrophic the disease (cancer, AIDS, etc.), the more likely there will be no appetite for food. The reason for this is obvious. When the body is sick it needs all the energy it can muster to heal itself. Since digestion requires so much energy, the appetite is shut down so available energy can be used for healing, not digestion.

When the body is fed lots of protein foods and simultaneously deprived of the carbohydrates it needs to carry out all the functions of life, two things happen. First, morning, noon and night the body is taxed and overworked by having to expend so much of its available energy converting the protein into the carbohydrates it needs. Second, the body, which essentially feels threatened because it doesn't have the fuel energy it needs to sustain itself, shuts down the appetite, as though it were sick, as it tries to conserve what energy it has. Weight is lost, but overall health progressively and steadily deteriorates because the body is consistently deprived of the one most important food for fuel: carbohydrates.

Even starches (pasta, bread, grains, etc.), which are at least already carbohydrates, unlike protein and fats, also have to go through a conversion process, because all starches are polysaccharides and can only be made available to the body (brain) in the form of glucose after they have been converted into monosaccharides. Again, an energy-intensive process.

Quiz time! Guess what one food in all the natural world is a monosaccharide without having to go through even the least bit of conversion to be so? Yes! That's right, fruit! A+ for you. The sugar in fruit, namely fructose (not porktose you notice), passes through the stomach and is absorbed through the walls of the intestines without undergoing any digestion. This leaves a great surplus of body energy available for living and all the activities that make living a joy. So not only does fruit *not require* any energy to be broken down, but it makes energy available faster and more efficiently than any other food in existence—an unbeatable combination.

In the vast array and variety of foods in the human diet, fruit stands entirely alone in its uniqueness. All foods—*all*—require time in the stomach for digestion. All except fruit.

The more quickly and efficiently food leaves the stomach the better. Why? Ever notice how tired you are after a big meal? Think back to last Thanksgiving. Ever hear of the afternoon siesta? The reason you feel tired after eating is because food in the stomach is a number-one priority in the body. The more you eat and the longer it has to stay in the stomach, the more energy you have to use and the more tired you will be.

Here's something you probably didn't know: Digestion requires more energy than anything else you can do. All the energy your body will use to digest the approximately seventy tons of food you will eat in this lifetime is more than all the energy you will expend for everything else in your lifetime *combined!* You don't have to have an IQ over 200 to figure out that anything you can do to optimize the efficiency of your digestive processes would be an extremely wise thing to do.

There are many ironies in this life we are all journeying through, and I can think of no other irony more bewildering than the one associated with the lack of high regard for the one food that most surely deserves it more than any other. Here is a line of reasoning that we may consider with profit: Whereas it follows that fruit, fulfilling the requirement for nutrients and energy more fully and perfectly than any other food, could reasonably be expected to comprise the bulk of our diet, does it not speak loudly to the abnormality of our Western diet that fruit is relegated to the last place on the menu as almost an afterthought, and is all too often used merely for ornamental purposes?

---

*Every society honors its live conformists
and its dead troublemakers.*

—Mignon McLaughlin

Here's another irony associated with fruit. Most people have no idea whatsoever that there is a right way and a wrong way to eat fruit, so they not only lose all the benefits it can provide, but they actually eat it in such a way as to cause harm. And as I stated earlier, learning the correct way to eat fruit has been the most important dietary lesson I (and millions of others) have ever learned.

Now, it's your turn. In order to reap the many benefits of fruit and change your life for the better in the process, there are two, let's call them guidelines, to acknowledge and adhere to. First, all fruit and fruit juice must be consumed in their natural state—not cooked, heated, processed, refined, pasteurized, irradiated or altered in any way. Second, because of fruit's unique nature in that it does not require time in the stomach for digestion, it should be consumed alone and on an empty stomach.

Now, as to the first, this book is about life, remember? It's about supplying your living body with living food. As pointed out in the chapter on living food versus dead food, heat kills. The life of any living thing on this planet, plant or animal, entirely depends upon the condition of its enzymes. If enzymes are intact, life continues. If enzymes are killed, life ceases. Remember that the heat to cook food is far in excess of what it takes to completely kill enzymes.

Eating fruit or drinking fruit juice that has been cooked or heated renders it not only valueless, but harmful.

You are perhaps familiar with the pH of your body, which refers to your body's acid–alkaline balance. On a scale of 0 to 14, zero represents pure acid, 14 represents pure alkaline, and 7 is neutral. The bloodstream is approximately 7.35 to 7.45 pH. In other words, our blood is slightly alkaline, and our health depends upon it remaining so. The leeway is very small. Even merely dipping below the neutral point of 7 into the acid range can be fatal. The standard American diet (SAD) is primarily acid-forming, which, you can be sure, is a major contributing factor to the poor health and overweight condition of the population.

As though fulfilling the two most important prerequisites of a food, that of supplying nutrients and energy for the body, were not enough, the specialness of fruit is further validated here. All fruit is alkaline and therefore neutralizes acid in the body. Whenever I mention that all fruit is alkaline, the first thing people say is, "What about oranges, grapefruits, pineapples and lemons? They're all acid fruits." True enough, but that is only their botanical classification. Once inside the body, all fruit is alkaline, *unless* it is subjected to heat, in which case it is acidic and contributes to the problems associated with a predominantly acid-producing diet. Once heated by any means, fruit and fruit juice go from being one of the primary tools in acquiring and maintaining a consistent level of good health to yet one more factor in the decline of well-being. This is nothing short of a tragedy, especially in light of the fact that, but for the lack of some simple education, this supreme gift of nature remains largely unknown and unutilized by most people.

Nothing illustrates this troublesome situation more strikingly than the circumstances that surround one of Nature's most perfect foods. The truest, most reliable test of all to determine the worthiness of *any* given food is to test it on babies. If an infant will fare well and thrive on it at a time when its growth and development are more crucial than at any other time in its life, you have a winner. The food I am referring to here is orange juice. It has been known for at least three-quarters of a century that babies whose mothers were, for some reason, unable to breast-feed could be fed on orange juice and they would flourish.[1]

I personally have known women who, for one reason or another, could not breast-feed at all, or who had no milk after a few days or a week. They fed their babies fresh-squeezed orange juice, and the children grew up strong and healthy without all the childhood afflictions that customarily plague children fed on formula, one of the most objectionable insults against life ever concocted (more on that later). Other juices were ultimately given, such as apple, grape and melon, but orange juice was the primary food. The key is, of course, that the juice was fresh, *not* pasteurized. Pasteurization subjects food to a heat so high that nothing living could possibly survive. So instead of the juice being living, vital and health-promoting, it is made to be dead, acidic and harmful.

For as long as I can remember, orange juice has been the symbol of the perfect morning drink. Orange juice is as commonplace on a breakfast table as a knife and fork. I grew up as one of five boys in a household where there was virtually no consciousness of eating healthfully. My folks were born and raised in Brooklyn, New York, in the early part of the 1900s and lived through wars, the Depression and hard times. "Good" food was whatever food could be put on the table. My mom, bless her sweet heart, repeated by rote the standard admonitions of the day, such as "eat your vegetables" and "drink your milk." But her one unwavering commitment to the health of her family was that everyone drink a big tumbler of orange juice every morning—"a glass of Florida sunshine," she called it.

All of us knew how to make the orange juice in the morning, and the job generally fell onto whomever was the first one in the kitchen. It was easy: You took one of the little cans of frozen concentrate out of the freezer, put the contents into a pitcher, added water and presto! Orange juice for everyone. I know my mom took great pride in doing this good thing for her family every morning. The only thing was that my mom and millions of other moms were and are to this very day the victims of one of the most successful and long-running cashectomies. You remember what a cashectomy is, right? It is being convinced to buy something advertised as good for you and winding up with something actually bad for you.

Nothing is so firmly believed as that which is least known.

—CHARLES AUGUSTIN MONTAIGNE

Orange juice made from concentrate is pasteurized. It's dead, acidic and harmful. The billion-dollar orange-juice industry is based on convincing you, the consumer, with every possible enticement to buy and drink orange juice. You're told how it's all-natural, how delicious it is, how packed with vitamin C and other nutrients it is, how good it is for you and your family, how it's Nature's gift to your well-being. And every word spoken about it would be true, *if it were not first destroyed by heat!*

It's not only concentrated orange juice that's pasteurized; most of those multicolored cartons and bottles of orange juice you see in grocery stores, with the many proclamations of all the goodness contained within, are one and all pasteurized, meaning they're denatured, devitalized and destructive. And it's not only orange juice, by the way. Apple, grape, cranberry, grapefruit, you name it, they're pasteurized. And more often than not they're laced with some refined sugar, additives, preservatives and other various and sundry chemicals. It's everything *but* natural.

Somehow the professional cashectomists have managed to obtain legislation that allows them to advertise and sell something as "all natural" when, after pasteurization, juice is no more natural than a hand grenade. Concerned and diligent parents all over this country, desirous of furnishing something for themselves and their children that is wholesome, nutritious and beneficial—exactly what the false advertisements declare it to be—are instead unwittingly serving up something unwholesome, unnutritious and hurtful.

How would you like to go to a jewelry store, buy and pay

for a beautiful diamond ring, then be given a rhinestone instead? You wouldn't care for that too much now, would you? At least a rhinestone can't acidify your blood and burn a hole in your stomach the way pasteurized fruit juice can.

Here's another little nugget of information you may find interesting. There is a frenetic preoccupation with taking calcium in this country. People have been whipped into a frenzy of fear over it. I'm going to discuss calcium a little later on, but for now it would be instructive for you to know that one of the primary functions of calcium in the body is to neutralize acid. If the diet is calcium-poor, the body leaches the calcium it needs from the bones and teeth and uses it instead. Even though our calcium needs can *easily* be supplied through diet, many people opt to take calcium supplements "just to be sure." Orange juice—fresh, unpasteurized orange juice, that is—is alkaline, so it helps neutralize acid in the body. But when it's pasteurized, not only do you lose its neutralizing effect and calcium-saving properties, but to make matters worse, it *adds* more acid to the body. Perhaps you can see why I describe the lack of understanding on this subject as a tragedy.

Experience tells me that there are those of you who are convinced you can't drink orange juice because you experience pain and discomfort whenever you do. I wish you could know the number of people I've encountered who thought that very thing until they started to drink it unpasteurized and on an empty stomach. I've known people who stopped drinking orange juice for more than fifteen years—it simply was not a part of their diet. Then upon learning this information, they reintroduced it in the proper way and now enjoy orange juice daily.

All of the possible negatives associated with fruit and fruit juices can be avoided, and all the potential benefits they have to offer can be fully realized, simply by consuming them the way God intended: unprocessed, unrefined, unheated, unchanged from their natural state. This first of the two guidelines on how to eat fruit correctly, which in turn plays a huge role in your quest to lose weight, cannot and should not be minimized. Now this is not to imply that you should never again have a piece of apple pie or drink a glass of cranberry-apple juice. I would never put a restriction on anyone to which I myself would not want to adhere. I'll tell you straight up, I love having a piece of apple pie (peach and blueberry, too) on occasion. And when I do, I enjoy it to the fullest degree. I simply acknowledge the fact that I'm eating it to satisfy myself on some emotional or psychological level. It's for my taste buds. I have it, I enjoy it, and I move on with no guilt or recriminations. The most important thing is that it comprises but a tiny percentage of the amount of fruit I eat overall, the preponderance of which is in its natural condition. I don't ever have pasteurized orange juice under any circumstance because I don't like the biting, acidic flavor of it, but I will on occasion have apple or grape juice that has been heated if it is all that is available at the time. This is my suggestion to you: Maintain the consciousness of striving as best you can to eat fruit and drink fruit juice in their natural state, and when you occasionally stray from that goal, forgive yourself and acknowledge the effort and commitment you *are* making to your well-being the majority of the time.

Most of our so-called reasoning consists in finding arguments for going on believing as we already do.

—JAMES ROBINSON

Here you might expect to hear that lame, tired, old cop-out of "everything in moderation." I can't stand that weak rationalization, invariably used by someone trying to convince you to use or buy something that is no good for you. Have you ever noticed that whenever someone says "everything in moderation" it's *always* in reference to something that does not promote health and that we can live perfectly well without? It's never "breathe fresh air in moderation," or "drink pure water in moderation," or "eat fresh wholesome food in moderation." No, what I'm talking about is being flexible, not fanatical. Whether it's politics, religion, relationships or diet, fanaticism does not work. Be flexible instead. It's what makes this a lifestyle, not a life sentence.

Before moving on to the second guideline for eating fruit correctly, I must dispel a long-standing myth that is based on nothing but ignorance. Some dietitians, nutritionists *and* medical doctors who never studied nutrition declare, in a way that might cause you to think they actually knew what they were talking about, that inside the body all sugars are the same, that all carbohydrates are the same, regardless of where they come from. Ordinarily, I wouldn't spend any time on such idiocy. However, some unwary folks who don't know any better, or who haven't had the opportunity to hear the nonfiction version, are actually being misled. They accept as valid the preposterous notion that there is no difference between how the body reacts to a candy bar and the way it reacts to a fresh piece of fruit—that drinking a Coca-Cola is the same as drinking fresh-squeezed orange juice. I personally have heard people who are referred to as "experts in the field" or "authorities on the subject" say this. It would be *exactly* like saying all liquids are the same when in contact with the body. Whether it's water or sulfuric acid, they're both liquids, so it makes no difference. Which would you rather have splashed on your skin?

Beware of false knowledge;
it is more dangerous than ignorance.

—GEORGE BERNARD SHAW

One reason why this absurd position is taken by those who have had their common-sense gene surgically removed is because the category of carbohydrates is so large. Pasta, bread, rice and other grains, cereals, pastries, potatoes, chips, sodas, candy—they're all classified as carbohydrates. So are fruit and vegetables. Remember, there are three major food groups: proteins, fats and carbohydrates. Fruit and fruit juices fall into the carbohydrate category, but there the similarities end, especially when they are consumed in their natural state. The idea of equating a highly processed, chemical-laden, intensely heated carbohydrate of any kind to a fresh piece of fruit or fruit juice is bizarre, laughable, ridiculous, absurd, crazy, beyond the pale . . . shall I go on? Can you tell that this particular subject makes the hair stand up on the back of my neck?

There is *one* thing that differentiates a fresh piece of fruit from all of the other processed carbohydrates mentioned above. That one thing is the heart of the message of this book: *life!* The life force that animates everything living exists; that is self-evident. Even though this life force can't be seen, you *know* it's there. You can't see electricity either, but is there any doubt in your mind that electricity exists? If you put a grain of wheat into the soil, it sprouts. If you heat the grain of wheat first, it won't sprout. Why? *Because it's dead.* Cooked to death. Even grains of wheat found in ancient tombs in Egypt, two thousand years old, will sprout if planted, but not if they are killed by cooking. Why is this simple, obvious fact of life so difficult for the so-called experts to grasp? Enzymes, the stuff of life, are killed when cooked.

It's not so much what folks don't know
that causes problems, it's what
they do know that ain't so.

—ARTEMUS WARD

No greater roadblock exists in bringing this life-enhancing awareness to the population than those experts, in name only, who wave their cherished credentials around and then open their mouths and prove that they have been educated beyond their intelligence. Although they can speak eloquently and seemingly knowledgeably, what they prove most clearly is that they know a whole lot about what isn't so. They ignore the obvious and obstinately hold on to the past because they can't allow themselves to admit they have spent their time being miseducated. I refer to them as the Nutritional Neanderthals who refuse to join us here in the twenty-first century.

While reading an article on the trend toward eating more living food for health, I was enormously encouraged to read a quote by Brian Clement, director of the Hippocrates Health Institute in West Palm Beach, Florida. Brian has been the nutritional consultant there for thirty years and has helped thousands of people from all over the world recapture their health after being given a death sentence by the medical community. I personally have recommended dozens of people go there, and they have been transformed.

I was filled with pride and hope when Brian stated that, "Raw food is now considered the number-one choice of serious health seekers, and the living food movement has begun to replace the vegetarian movement, a transformation that will be complete in ten to fifteen years."[2]

The article also had a quote from an R.D., L.D./N., that's Registered Dietitian and Licensed Dietitian/Nutritionist. Whew, there's a mouthful of credentials for you. But they left off N.N.—Nutritional Neanderthal. In this person's own words, "Enzymes are proteins. We digest the protein from food whether it's raw or cooked." Poor thing. She has the classical, inexplicable blind spot that prevents her from realizing that digesting is only half the story. What is digested must be assimilated by the body or it's worthless. The living body wants living food, not dead food. It's a good thing people can't be jailed for blind ignorance or I'm afraid this R.D., L.D./N., N.N. would never again see the light of day.

Trust in this, for it will serve you well for the rest of your life: Fresh fruit and fruit juices are living and thereby able to release and provide all the goodness that life has to offer—*if* they are consumed correctly. Since you now know the first guideline for eating fruit correctly, unheated and in its natural state, let's move on to the second guideline.

Recall, if you will, the exceedingly important revelation made earlier, that fruit stands alone as the one and only food in the entire food chain that requires no digestion in the stomach. No digestive enzymes have to be produced by the body (as have to be with other foods) because all the enzymes required for digestion are already in the fruit as long as they are not destroyed by heat. This unique feature means that in order for fruit to be properly broken down and utilized effectively, it is essential that all fruit be allowed to pass through the stomach to the intestines unimpeded so its full potential can be realized. The only way to stop it on its journey through the stomach is if there is already food in the stomach or if the fruit is eaten along with food that must stay in the stomach. When this happens and fruit comes into contact with digestive juices, it spoils and turns to acid. All the positives associated with eating fruit correctly are lost and turned into negatives. It causes starches to ferment and proteins to putrefy, which in turn causes so many of the digestive disorders that are so prevalent. Billions upon billions of dollars are spent every year to treat acid indigestion and other digestive ailments. I'm not saying that eating fruit incorrectly is the sole cause, not by a long shot, but there can be no doubt that it contributes significantly to the problem.

It is always easier to believe than to deny.
Our minds are naturally affirmative.

—JOHN BURROUGHS

The way people react to new information varies greatly from person to person, especially when it's completely and totally brand-new. I have watched these reactions with great enjoyment over the years. At that instant when the realization first hits people that fruit has a certain correct way of being eaten and they have been doing the opposite their entire lives, every range of emotion can be experienced. Some people open their eyes as wide as saucers. Others drop their jaws onto their chests. Some pretend to hit themselves in the head with the heel of their hands, while others express themselves verbally with something like, "Oh man, I can't believe it." Some people exhibit frustration or exasperation, while others actually become angry that they had never heard a word of it before. People let out deep sighs, whistle, roll their eyes or moan.

It's most interesting to me when I share this information with an audience at seminars. It never fails, as I look around the room I see it all unfold before my eyes—people poking each other and making comments and facial expressions. Invariably people come up to me afterwards with their experiences, their "war stories," that they feel a strong need to share. Most are relieved to finally have an answer to why they feel the way they do when all their doctors could ever tell them was, "You have a sensitive stomach; take an antacid."

I mean it when I say I could fill this book with comments and stories people have shared with me. I already told you of the many instances of people discovering that orange juice can actually be enjoyed without pain. I'm not going to load you up with a bunch of testimonials here, but there are two quick ones I'd like to share because they stand out in my mind.

The first is a woman who was taken to a carnival as a little girl where, after eating a hot dog, she had a bowl of strawberries. She had a violent reaction. Her skin became hot and flushed, and she was in considerable pain. Her mother took her to the hospital, where she was informed by the doctor that she was allergic to strawberries. No mention was made of the hot dog, made of who-knows-what, wrapped in a white-flour bun. The perceived villain was the strawberries. From that day forward, although she had a natural attraction to strawberries, she had in her mind that she had some kind of allergy that was out of her control. Whenever the attraction was too strong to ignore, she would have the berries she so desired and, sure enough, she would experience some type of discomfort. She would have them after a meal, on cereal, or in strawberry shortcake or strawberry pie or strawberries and cream. The only way she did *not* have them was alone and on an empty stomach. As a grown woman, a friend of hers brought her to one of my seminars, and the effect on her upon hearing the correct way of eating strawberries was like having a piano dropped on her. She subsequently came to another seminar and related to me her story and the delight she now has at eating strawberries with no pain and discomfort.

People should think things out fresh and not just accept conventional terms and the conventional way of doing things.

—BUCKMINSTER FULLER

Sometimes I'll be on stage and see people in the audience having a very animated reaction to what they are learning, and I just *know* they are going to come up and tell me their tales. Such was the case when I saw a woman in one of the first few rows who was obviously having an epiphany as the revelation of what she had been doing incorrectly swept over her. Sure enough, she waited patiently for the crowd of people that inevitably forms around a speaker after a talk to disperse. She was practically in tears of joy. You see, she loved melons, especially honeydew melons. She found chilled melon to be the perfect after-dinner treat to wash the palate and refresh the mouth. The only thing is, it invariably made her "gassy," in addition to the fact that she would find herself "burping it up all night," which she found annoying to say the least. She had gotten to the point where she thought she would just have to forgo eating melons. As it happens, I used as an example in the seminar a man who loved honeydew but always burped it up all night. I stated the guideline governing correct fruit eating and said that if the honeydew was eaten first, on an empty stomach, it would never be heard from again. When she heard this she just about fell out of her seat. I received a letter from her a few weeks later wherein she went on and on about how thrilled she was to have found this information that has helped her so much—long overdue, to be sure, but welcomed nonetheless. Another satisfied customer.

Fruit for dessert is a way of life in our culture, and here I am tearing it down and describing it as a destructive habit that compromises your health. There are those who express shock, even disbelief that the habit would continue to be so popular if it is as detrimental as I suggest. But actually it's not hard at all to see that something hurtful can go on for years—even centuries—and not be recognized as such until something comes along that proves itself to be more reliable and advantageous. After all, look how long we have been cooking all the life out of our food and trying to survive on it instead of consuming the living food the living body requires.

There are those, surely, who eat fruit incorrectly and don't experience any discomfort whatsoever. I know that.

Not everyone does. There are some people with iron-clad stomachs who can eat lightbulbs, with or without fruit, and feel nothing. But they are the minority. Someone is shelling out billions of dollars for digestive aids. Besides, even if no discomfort is felt, what is of greatest importance is that fruit be allowed to pass through the stomach unhindered so as to avoid all possible harm while providing all the potential benefits it has to offer.

Knowing what I do about eating fruit the correct way, when I see someone eating a piece of honeydew wrapped in fancy ham or some other indiscretion, it is like listening to someone scratch a blackboard with her fingernails. I just want to get right up in the person's face and say, "Hey, do you have any idea what you're doing there?" I don't, but believe it or not, I used to. When I first learned about it and experienced success in doing it right, I was young and unsophisticated to say the least. I would go up to complete strangers and start reading them the riot act. This, of course, was met with mixed reactions. As odd as it might sound, most people were quite civil about my accosting them. Some were surprised, even shocked, to hear what I told them, and some were actually grateful that I took the time to talk to them. Others were neutral and said, "Thanks, but no thanks," while others simply called security on me. As you might imagine, this made me a highly sought-after guest at dinner parties. After all, what host or hostess would not want to have in attendance someone telling the other dinner guests that the food being served to them was contributing to their demise?

READER/CUSTOMER CARE SURVEY

We care about your opinions. Please take a moment to fill out this Reader Survey card and mail it back to us.

As a special "thank you" we'll send you exciting news about interesting books and a valuable **Gift Certificate.**

Please PRINT using ALL CAPS

First Name [   ]   MI. [ ]   Last Name [   ]

Address [   ]

City [   ]   ST [   ]   Zip [   ] — [   ]

Phone # ([   ]) [   ] — [   ]   Fax # ([   ]) [   ] — [   ]

Email [   ]

(1) Gender:
___ Female   ___ Male

(2) Age:
___ 12 or under   ___ 40-59
___ 13-19   ___ 60+
___ 20-39

(3) Marital Status
___ Married
___ Single
___ Divorced/Widowed

(4) Did you receive this book as a gift?
___ Yes   ___ No

(5) How many Health Communications books have you bought or read?
___ 1   ___ 2-4   ___ 5+
.

(6) How did you find out about this book?
Please fill in ONE.
1) ___ Recommendation
2) ___ Store Display
3) ___ Bestseller List
4) ___ Online
5) ___ Advertisement
6) ___ Catalog/Mailing
7) ___ Interview/Review (TV, Radio, Print)

(7) Where do you usually buy books?
Please fill in your top TWO choices.
1) ___ Bookstore
2) ___ Religious Bookstore
3) ___ Online
4) ___ Book Club/Mail Order
5) ___ Price Club (Costco, Sam's Club, etc.)
6) ___ Retail Store (Target, Wal-Mart, etc.)

(9) What subjects do you enjoy reading about most? Rank only FIVE. Use 1 for your favorite, 2 for second favorite, etc.

	1	2	3	4	5
1) Parenting/Family	O	O	O	O	O
2) Relationships	O	O	O	O	O
3) Recovery/Addictions	O	O	O	O	O
4) Health/Nutrition	O	O	O	O	O
5) Christianity	O	O	O	O	O
6) Spirituality/Inspiration	O	O	O	O	O
7) Business Self-Help	O	O	O	O	O
8) Teen Issues	O	O	O	O	O
9) Sports	O	O	O	O	O

(14) What attracts you most to a book?
(Please rank 1-4 in order of preference.)

	1	2	3	4
1) Title	O	O	O	O
2) Cover Design	O	O	O	O
3) Author	O	O	O	O

TAPE IN MIDDLE; DO NOT STAPLE

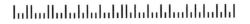

FOLD HERE

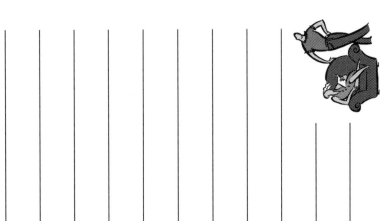

Comments:

> Crank—a person with a new
> idea until it succeeds.
>
> —MARK TWAIN

There's a very good reason why this section on fruit is the longest section in the book. That is because it can have, more than anything else, the greatest impact on your success. If you can, at least temporarily, set aside all your preconceived notions of what and when to eat; if you can suspend your present beliefs, only momentarily, as to what you have been taught is the optimum way to eat; if you can commit to an admittedly revolutionary approach to eating, only as a test to see if it has merit; if you can clear your mind of all of it and just trust that you have come into possession of this book because it has some of the answers you have been searching for; then you, like hundreds of thousands before you, will see that there is a way to eat, and eat the foods you like, and still be able to lose weight and maintain a high level of health.

Consider the old adage, "The greater the risk, the greater the reward." Not that I'm asking you to risk anything, but I am going to ask you to take a leap of faith with what I am about to suggest to you as regards how to eat more fruit and eat it correctly. I know from experience that what I'm about to recommend will be, for some of you—not all, but definitely some of you—a tremendous challenge. There's no sense in pretending it won't be. But on the other side, it will also produce the greatest reward. You see, I'm not just asking you to continue with your present eating habits and merely start eating fruit correctly. No. It is important, in fact essential, that fruit play a more significant role in your diet and that it comprise a greater amount of your overall food intake than it does at present.

Who dares nothing, need hope for nothing.

—JOHANN VON SCHILLER

I can tell you that what I'm about to propose is not based on a whim or a guess that it will work. It's not an arbitrary experiment featuring you as the test subject. It's not trial and error. It has proven highly effective for a great number of people over a very long period of time. Yes, it is most definitely different from what you've been accustomed to, but that is precisely what is needed considering that what has been employed to date has not done the job.

By way of introducing what will likely be a brand-new concept to you (unless you are familiar with my previous books), I am going to acquaint you with a most interesting aspect of your own body with which you might be unfamiliar. You have probably heard mention of your body cycles, or what are referred to as circadian rhythms. Circadian refers to the regular recurrence of cycles of activity that occur every twenty-four hours. All biological activities occur at regular intervals regardless of other conditions such as constant darkness or light.

There are three activities associated with eating and turning food into body-cell structure. They could not be more obvious. We eat food, the body extracts what it needs from the food, and the residue is eliminated. The three cycles are referred to as the appropriation cycle (eating), the assimilation cycle (extraction of nutrients) and the elimination cycle (elimination of wastes). Without question, all three cycles are ongoing twenty-four hours a day, but each has its own eight-hour cycle during which its activities are most heightened. The appropriation cycle is from 12:00 noon until 8:00 P.M. This is when the body is most capable of efficiently taking in and digesting food. The assimilation cycle is from 8:00 P.M. to 4:00 A.M. During the hours of sleep, the body is extracting what it needs. The elimination cycle is from 4:00 A.M. to 12:00 noon. The body is gathering wastes and preparing them for removal.

It is the elimination cycle on which we need to focus our attention. If you want to lose weight, you wish to eliminate the excess from your body, do you not? One thing I can assure you of with the same certainty I would that the sun is hot and a glacier is cold is that the probability of you successfully losing weight is immensely enhanced when your elimination cycle is freed up to function at its optimum efficiency. Of this there is absolutely no doubt.

When I talk about your elimination cycle, I am not merely talking about waking up in the morning and having a bowel movement. It is so very, *very* much more than that. Every last one of the 100 trillion cells in your body is in itself a small, extremely active and dynamic processing plant. Each one is taking in the nutrients it needs, performing literally tens of thousands of life functions and producing its own waste that must be eliminated. So important is the removal of this waste that the most extensive system in the human body, the lymph system, has as its primary function the task of collecting all the wastes from every cell, degrading the waste—breaking it down—and preparing it for removal from one of the four eliminative organs of the body: the bowels, bladder, lungs and skin. I will be discussing the lymph system in more detail later, but for now, you should know that there is *three times* more lymph fluid in your body than there is blood,[3] which should give you some sense of the extremely important role the lymph system plays in the elimination of wastes from your body. If the lymph system is overburdened or if the elimination cycle is prevented from operating at its highest level, successful weight loss is problematic, to put it mildly. It has been my experience over the last three decades that the people in most need of losing weight are dealing with both. That is, their lymph systems are bogged down, and the activities of their elimination cycle are severely diminished. Let me tell you, if weight loss is your goal, that's a bad combination. The reason you are now going to be successful in your quest to lose weight is that the three Keys to Success are designed *specifically* to optimize the effectiveness of both your lymph system and your elimination cycle.

It is not at all an exaggeration to state that having a grasp of the vital role your elimination cycle plays in every area of your well-being, and doing what is necessary to assist it in that effort, is one of, if not the most, important bits of knowledge you will ever learn in regards to your health. It is indeed a sorrowful commentary that an understanding of this integral component of a healthy life is so completely unknown that there are millions of people, young and old, whose elimination cycles have not been given the opportunity to function freely, uninterrupted, for even one single day of their lives. *Not one.* Anything you are currently doing, knowingly or not, that is hindering your elimination cycle is something you need to *stop* doing. Anything you can do to assist or further improve your elimination cycle is something you need to *start* doing. As it happens, what I'm about to ask you to do succeeds in accomplishing *both* simultaneously.

What is it then that impedes the elimination cycle, preventing it from operating at its highest capacity? We know that every activity of the body, large or small, requires energy. Whether blinking your eyes or climbing a flight of stairs, every activity of the body requires some of the finite amount of energy it has on hand. The brain prioritizes and portions out this available energy where it is needed. Recall, if you will, what activity is the number-one priority, requiring more energy than all other expenditures of energy combined. Digestion! Of necessity, the elimination cycle, indeed *every* system of the body, has to relinquish some of the energy allocated to its efforts and share it with the digestive system in order to deal with the number-one priority of food in the stomach—unless, of course, that food happens to be fruit, which, as you know, does not require any digestive energy.

Every public action, which is not
customary, either is wrong, or, if it is right,
is a dangerous precedent. It follows
that nothing should ever be
done for the first time.

—FRANCES CORNFORD

Here then is what I'm asking you to do, which I have said is the single most important thing I have ever learned about health and is the factor more responsible for my own recaptured well-being than any other. From the time you wake up in the morning until noon, put nothing into your stomach other than fruit and fruit juice. That's it. Oh, I can hear the howls. "What?! No breakfast? Are you nuts? You gotta be kidding." For those of you who are about to slam this book shut and make some further crack about my sanity, please calm down and take a breath. I know that for you who are convinced that "breakfast is the most important meal of the day" or who simply look forward to and enjoy breakfast, I have crossed the line. I understand. When I was first told in 1970 how crucial this was for me to lose weight and improve my health, I was, to put it mildly, displeased. Stunned was more like it. "Oh no," I said, "not that. Breakfast is one of my three favorite times of day to eat."

Actually, the comments I have heard from people hearing this suggestion for the first time range anywhere from, "Wow, that's great, this is going to be a cinch for me. I've never really been attracted to big meals in the morning and only had them because I was told it was best," to, "No, no, please don't tell me that. I'd rather be hit in the face with a battle ax than not eat breakfast." And everything in between.

First, let me state that I'm not saying *no* breakfast. I'm saying a healthful breakfast is different from what you may be accustomed to eating. Second, let's look at the reasoning behind what may first appear to be so radical a position. The appropriation cycle, which is from noon to 8:00 P.M., is when the body is predisposed to digest food and will allot the energy to do so. It follows that after the food has been digested, energy will then be allocated to extract and utilize the nutrients it needs and will be followed by the elimination of what is not used. To force the appropriation cycle into action *prior* to the completion of the elimination cycle not only severely retards the process of accumulating wastes from the body, it also throws the rhythm of the three cycles into turmoil.

When you awaken in the morning, sometime between 4:00 A.M. and 12:00 noon, the elimination cycle is in full swing, at its highest activity level—the *exact opposite* of the appropriation cycle, which is, in fact, dormant. That is by design. The intelligence of the body has worked it out so that the one activity of the body that requires more energy than any other, digestion, is at rest, requiring *no* energy so that the elimination cycle will not be disrupted. The very moment food enters the stomach requiring digestion, energy *must* be allocated to deal with it, and the elimination cycle suffers a loss of some of the energy that was being used to perform the vital task of waste removal. Fruit requires no digestion in the stomach. You can eat all the fruit you want, any time you want, correctly of course, and the elimination cycle will not be affected in the least.

Even though this business of the cycles is something you are perhaps unfamiliar with, and you are unaccustomed to the idea of fruit only until noon, the more you think about it, the more sense it will make.

Much of the wisdom of one age
is the folly of the next.

—CHARLES SIMMONS

History is teeming with examples of ideas that were at first judged to be so revolutionary, so devoid of worthiness, they were rejected out-of-hand without so much as a cursory hearing, only to become standard practice once their true value became undeniable.

When it was first suggested that physicians wash their hands before surgery, the proponent of this suggestion, Ignaz Semmelweis, was ridiculed and literally laughed out of his chosen profession.

In the mid-1800s, cool water was withheld from fever patients because it was actually believed—in fact, it was "known"—to be harmful. Children whose throats were too raw to even talk would *plead* for a drink of water and be denied right up until death. Occasionally, when all hope of survival was gone, as a dying wish, water was given and the patient would recover. But still the belief was so strong that water was injurious to a fever patient that it was withheld, believing that cool water was "desperate bad for sick folks." One doctor of the day, whose brain stem was still attached, wanted to know, "Why it was that anything so good for well folks should be so bad for sick folks."[4]

In the early 1900s, heart attacks were becoming more and more common. They were so grossly misunderstood at the time that physical activity was discouraged as it would make the heart wear out. Instead, cardiology patients were forced to lie flat on their backs for six weeks with as little movement as possible. In 1924, Dr. Paul Dudley White, "the father of cardiology," founded the American Heart Association. He stunned the medical world when he insisted that heart-attack patients get up and start a daily walking routine as soon as possible. Not only was his advice shunned and ridiculed at the time, but it was another *thirty years* before it was acknowledged and accepted as the best way to treat a patient after a heart attack.[5]

In each of these three examples, what was first ridiculed and thought to be unworthy of serious consideration came to be standard operating procedure. Dozens and dozens more examples could be given in every area of life. I'm not naive; I know there will be those who will cling to the past and obstinately insist we continue doing what we have been doing all along, even though nothing could be more obvious that some change in what we have been doing is necessary. I only pray it's not another thirty years before the understanding of what constitutes the proper and best food to eat in the morning hours is accepted and given the credit it deserves.

Let's quickly do away with another myth. Ever heard this one? "You have to eat a hearty breakfast for energy." Nothing could be more absurd. It would be like saying I have to jump in a pool of water to dry off, or I have to drink a bottle of whiskey to sober up. The digestion of food *requires* energy. Food will remain in your stomach for about three hours before it ever passes into your intestines, where the process of extracting what is needed to build up a storehouse of energy can begin. That's why you are tired after eating a big meal, not energized. It's all so obvious. When you go to sleep at night "dead tired" and wake up in the morning renewed, it wasn't because you ate, it was because your body built up its energy reserves for the next day while you slept. That's where energy comes from; it's built up while you sleep. It takes hours and hours for food to be transformed into energy. The very idea that you can eat a big meal of primarily cooked food that will provide usable energy shortly thereafter is laughable. Why do you think people eat "hearty breakfasts" and then start gulping down coffee and sodas for the caffeine lift?

One of the first, most immediate results people notice upon eating only fruit in the morning is the dramatic increase in their energy level. You know why? Because instead of the body *using up* energy to digest a meal, the sugar component in fruit, which you learned earlier is already a monosaccharide (meaning it turns to glucose with little or no effort from the body), is available as energy in the bloodstream quickly.

There are those people who may be thinking, *I have to go to work. If I don't eat, I won't have any energy.* You can rest assured that energy will be in far greater supply by eating a breakfast that requires no digestive energy than one that requires an abundance of digestive energy to be used. Plus, the fuel energy that you require to see you through the day will be in a purer form and more readily available from fruit than from any other food you can eat.

An expert is one who knows more
and more about less and less.

—NICHOLAS BUTLER

There's nothing easier to find than two people with opposite points of view. No matter what the subject, you can always find two people to disagree with one another. Turn on talk shows on the radio or TV and there will be no shortage of discussions, arguments and debates from people whose opinions differ entirely. Whatever your most strongly held beliefs are, the ones you would not give up without a fight, you can be sure there is someone, somewhere, who believes the exact opposite just as strongly. As fervently convinced as I am that eating only fruit until noon is the single greatest action you can take to further your health goals, I know, without a doubt, there is someone equally convinced that sausage and eggs are the way to go.

There are many truths of which the full
meaning cannot be realized until personal
experience has brought it home.

—JOHN STUART MILL

I'm going to stop right now trying to convince you of the
wisdom of eating only fruit until noon. It's not something
that can be proven with words, no matter how convincing
they are. Opinions and beliefs may differ, they may come
and go, but nothing can take the place of experience.
Experiencing a thing through personal verification is the
greatest teacher, the most accurate guide in determining
your attitude toward any given subject.

I'm going to show you how to prove it to yourself with a
simple, straightforward, easy-to-do test. As someone who
spent years in frustration before finding what worked, I
know what it's like to go on a diet for a month or two and
not wind up with the desired results. If your journey has
been long, then you know what I'm talking about. I'm not
going to ask you to do this for a month. You can have all
the proof you'll ever need in one week. One week from
today you will know exactly whether or not what I'm saying about fruit until noon is accurate. If you *have* been long
in your searching, then I would think that one week would
be very little to ask.

Here is what you do: Starting tomorrow morning from
the time you wake up until at least noon, consume nothing
but fresh-squeezed fruit juice and fresh fruit. You can have

as much as you like, as often as you like. If a small amount holds you, fine. If you want something every half hour, fine. No limits. Any type of fruit or juice works. The one hard-and-fast rule you commit to is only fruit and juice and absolutely nothing else. The one and only exception is if you want to drink water, which is, of course, fine also. You would be better off having nothing than to have fruit from a can or juice that has been pasteurized. Only fruit, only fresh and only for one week, seven days. Make no other changes whatsoever, none! From noon on, eat whatever you would normally eat. This way, at the end of the week, whatever changes you see you can be certain will be from the exclusive eating of only fruit and fruit juice before noon. On the eighth day, eat a big, hearty breakfast. Eat whatever breakfast you would normally have. It would be best if the eighth day is a day when you can lie around and nap—you'll need to.

In making this challenge I almost feel as though I'm cheating in that I already know the result. It would be like someone knowing who was going to win the World Series, and then betting on that team. I can't lose. The reason I am so certain is because of what I told you earlier about the hundreds of thousands of letters I've received from people all over the world. I told you that the greatest number of comments were about the effects of eating fruit correctly. I didn't relate precisely what was said because I had not yet introduced the concept of fruit only until noon. Now that I have, I can tell you that the comments were all about the benefits that were realized as a result of having only fruit until noon. Over and over again I read, "fruit 'til noon has changed my life." "At first it was a challenge, but now I could not imagine having anything but fruit 'til noon." "As years go by, I may waver in my discipline as to some aspects of my diet, but the one thing I do religiously is eat only fruit 'til noon." "Fruit in the morning has been a godsend for me." To this day, people come up and relate the same experience time and again.

Life is about becoming
more than we are.

—OPRAH WINFREY

I don't wish to belabor the point, but I am compelled to share one testimonial that stands out most clearly in my memory. It's been said that no fiction could ever rival the truth, that the truth is frequently stranger than fiction. So it is here. I couldn't have made up a story to serve as a grander testimony of the effect of eating only fruit until noon. It concerns a couple in their late thirties with two young children. The parents, Michael and Barbara, were both raised on a farm and brought up with the habit of socking down a "good ol' country breakfast" every morning. Both were in reasonably good health. They had their complaints, the standard stuff, a little overweight, headaches, colds, a desire for more energy since he went to work every day and she had her hands full with two young kids, but nothing really serious. Both made time to exercise every day, and they ate the standard American diet, including a big breakfast, meat and potatoes, and fast food on the weekends for the kids—which meant Mom didn't have to cook. They weren't the picture of health, but they didn't have one foot in the grave either.

Barbara was convinced to attend one of my seminars in Los Angeles by a friend of hers who had had some spectacular results with *Fit for Life*. At first, because it was all so new to her, she was rather overwhelmed because what I was recommending was so different from what she was accustomed to doing. She was, however, considerably intrigued with the idea of eating only fruit in the morning based solely on the fact that it made sense. She always ate a good-sized breakfast, but she was already starting to wonder if it wasn't the reason why she was always so tired all through the morning and afternoon. She decided to give it the one-week test and discussed it with her husband in the hopes he would do it with her. Michael was adamantly against it. Not that he was belligerent about it—he wasn't. He was devoted to his wife, respected her decision to try any dietary changes she wished and supported her completely in whatever decisions she made about her own life. But he wasn't about to give up the breakfasts he enjoyed in the morning. No way, no how.

After the one-week test, Barbara was blown away— dumbfounded—by the phenomenal increase in her energy level. After eating a heavy breakfast on the eighth day, following seven days of fruit and fruit juice only in the morning, she was a convert. She again appealed to her husband to just *try* it, based on her success and enthusiasm. Her entreaties fell on deaf ears. He was genuinely happy that

Barbara found something she was so thrilled about, but he wasn't interested. So when her family sat down to bacon and eggs or pancakes in the morning, she had a big fruit salad or a fruit smoothie, and everyone was happy.

Over the next three or four months, based on the success she had with fruit 'til noon, Barbara also started to use the other principle involved with incorporating more living food in the diet (which you will learn more about in the next chapter). Her life was transformed. She lost all the weight she had been wrestling with (on and off) for years, about seventeen pounds. Her energy level was supreme, her outlook on life was upbeat and positive, the little aches and pains she sometimes experienced disappeared, her skin cleared up and took on a glow she had not known for years, her hair was more lustrous, and her nails became stronger. She was like a poster child for this approach to eating. Obviously, Michael could not help but notice this transformation and started giving consideration to making the same changes Barbara had made. One morning the older of their two children asked, "Can I have just fruit for breakfast today?" That was it. Michael started doing everything to the letter that his wife was doing—and wouldn't you know it, his results were equally as remarkable. Lost weight, more energy, less pain, better attitude, everything.

Even their kids, accustomed to eating those horrid breakfast cereals that the cashectomists tease them with on TV until they nag their parents into buying them, started to change and eat more healthfully.

I met the entire family, and their rosy-cheeked exuberance for life was clearly tangible. You couldn't miss it; it was like a glow that surrounded them. It was, and is to this day, for me, one of the most gratifying illustrations of the value of the work I've dedicated myself to learning and sharing with the world.

Having shared this information with so many people for so long, I know there are questions that those who want to try fruit 'til noon have on their minds. Over the years I've been asked these questions so frequently that I pretty much know what you want to ask, so I'm going to end this chapter with a quick overview and some tips on how to make it more successful.

Tips and Hints for Eating Fruit 'til Noon

1. When first awakening in the morning, it is beneficial to drink a glass of water to wash through the digestive tract. This can have a squeeze of lemon in it or not.

2. All fruit and fruit juice must be fresh. Nothing cooked, canned or processed in any way. Nothing pasteurized.

3. You can have as much or as little as you desire up until noon. Some people are fine with only a small amount of fruit and desire no more. Others want to "graze" all morning on different fruits and juice. Either is fine. Figure out what is best for you and do that.

4. Fruits such as bananas, raisins, dates and all dried fruits (figs, pineapple, mango, papaya, apples, apricots) are more concentrated and will stay in your stomach longer than the watery fruits, so you will feel full longer. It is essential, however, to *not* eat fruit dried with chemicals such as sulfur nitrite. Eat *only*

naturally dried fruit. It will say on the package if it is sun-dried or dehydrated or if it contains sulfur nitrite, or your grocer will be able to tell you. Health-food stores usually have naturally dried fruit. Also food dehydrators have become popular as of late. They are inexpensive and valuable far beyond their cost. Since dried fruit is concentrated versus fresh fruit, which has a higher water content, it is extremely important that you only eat very small amounts of dried fruit. The bulk of what you eat should be the high-water-content fruits. As you know, you may have as much fresh fruit as you desire, but dried fruit, unlike fresh fruit, can be overeaten.

5. Some people want to know if it's all right to have nothing in the morning except water. Yes. What you are trying to do is not interfere with the elimination cycle with food that requires digestion. But unless you are one of the minuscule number of people who simply do not like to eat fruit, it is important that you eat some fruit every day, and in the morning is when you can be sure there is nothing else in the stomach that will cause fruit to spoil.

6. After drinking juice, which is primarily water, you can eat other foods after about ten to fifteen minutes have elapsed. After eating whole fruit or a smoothie [see next page], wait about thirty to forty minutes before eating other food. After eating bananas, raisins or dried fruit, you should wait about forty minutes. *Once you have eaten something other than fruit, you should wait at least three hours before eating fruit or*

drinking juice again. The only exception to this is that if you have raw vegetables by themselves without dressing or dip, fruit can then be eaten about twenty to thirty minutes later. If you wish to have fruit as a snack or at night before bed, be sure that at least three hours elapse after eating anything cooked and about one and a half to two hours after eating a salad.

A smoothie is made by putting into a blender chunks of frozen bananas (freeze peeled bananas in an air-tight container), fresh apple or orange juice, and whatever fresh or frozen fruit you like, such as strawberries, blueberries or other berries, peaches, etc. It blends into a delicious shake. Its thickness depends on the amount of bananas used. Some people like the bananas at room temperature—it's just a matter of taste. Experiment with these; they are delicious and fun. A day rarely passes that I don't have one of these treats.

7. Whenever drinking juice (or a smoothie), it is extremely important that you do not gulp it down. It should be consumed slowly. Drinking a glass of orange juice in two big gulps is not good for you and can cause your stomach to become upset. Take only one mouthful. Swish it around in your mouth one time to mix it with saliva and then swallow. In other words, "chew" your juice. This is not a small matter. *Drink your juices slowly; do not gulp them down.*

8. The question often comes up if it is all right to continue having juice after noon, or whether it is necessary to eat something else at twelve o'clock.

No, it is not necessary to eat something other than fruit at noon, unless you are hungry for something else. Many people, myself included, on numerous occasions have only fruit and fruit juice until the evening meal. Sometimes you simply won't feel like eating anything other than fruit, and you should not feel you must eat if you are not hungry. As you progress with this, there will even be days when you have only fruit and fruit juice the entire day. It's a totally natural thing; sometimes you just won't feel like eating. Those are truly super-high-energy days. As time goes by, and you become more familiar with eating fruit correctly, you will find there are a multitude of ways to provide your body with fruit. It's something that automatically happens and becomes clear to you over time. For now you should focus on having fruit exclusively 'til noon, and the rest will unfold and become familiar to you as a natural progression.

9. Something you will notice once you start having fruit 'til noon and more fruit in your diet in general is that you will urinate more frequently, and the color will range from cloudy to clear as water. This is a good thing. A *very* good thing. The high water content and cleansing properties of fruit will start to flush your body of toxins, and I can think of no greater gift to yourself than that. We are conditioned in this country to view with suspicion any change in our body's activities. People are actually made to fear certain bodily functions when they are out of the

"norm," as though the dynamic human body is ever static rather than constantly in a state of action and change. I know there are those who have been told that frequent urination can be a sign of diabetes. In certain circumstances that is true, but this is not one of them. The addition of more living food into your diet, especially the addition of more fruit and juice, *necessitates* more frequent urination.

10. There have been occasions when some people would tell me that although they are attracted to eating fruit, they are unable to do so because of the effect it has on them. They report that if they so much as eat an apple, their stomachs hurt and they get diarrhea. Of course, the fruit is blamed for this undesirable condition, and they therefore do not eat fruit. Invariably, this unwanted reaction to fruit is the result of a system so silted up with toxins that as soon as fruit, which is very cleansing, hits the intestines, it goes to work to clean it out. The diarrhea is the body's way of trying to clean and protect itself. It has been my experience that those who see it through and continue to eat a cleansing, predominantly living-food diet, with fruit as an integral part, will soon flush their bodies of these toxins and be able to eat fruit with no difficulty. It may take two or three days or even a week of some discomfort, but on the other side of it, the person who stays the course will feel renewed and be able to enjoy Nature's grandest culinary gift.

11. As the understanding of the three body cycles, and

the wisdom of allowing each eight-hour cycle to perform its intended role unhindered, deepens, a question is likely to arise as it has with so many others. It is this: Since we don't want to interfere with the elimination cycle by eating before noon, would it not also be wise to refrain from extending the appropriation cycle beyond 8:00 P.M. into the assimilation cycle? Should we not eat past 8:00 P.M.? As a general guideline, that is correct. I have found personally the best time to eat the evening meal is during the hour from 6:00 P.M. to 7:00 P.M. Later in the evening if you want to eat something, have fruit again before going to sleep because in the same way fruit does not interfere with the elimination cycle it doesn't take energy from the assimilation cycle. Remember to wait at least three hours to eat fruit after you've eaten a cooked meal. Eating cooked food at night and then going to sleep forces the body to expend energy on digestion during the time you would be sleeping. This is a prime reason why many people wake up groggy in the morning. Can you see if you eat late at night and then wake up in the morning and eat again, it's no wonder that so many people are chronically fatigued? There are other reasons for chronic fatigue syndrome, which I will address later, but I know several people who were diagnosed with chronic fatigue syndrome who were given drugs (gee, what a surprise) and told to go home and get more rest. As soon as they stopped eating cooked food during their elimination and assimilation cycles, their chronic fatigue syndrome "magically" went away. This is no joke; hundreds of thousands of people suffer from this disorder for no other reason than that they are interfering with their body's natural body cycles.

12. I'm often surprised how frequently people will express nervousness over eating more fruits and vegetables because of pesticides. Of all the toxic chemical residues found in the food consumed by Americans, less than 10 percent comes from fruits and vegetables. Over 90 percent comes from animal products. Factory farm animals have a dangerously high concentration of these chemical toxins in their bodies from a lifetime of eating feed that has been saturated with these deadly biocides. Never does anyone ever raise the question of pesticides in meat, chicken, fish, eggs or dairy, and that is where 90 percent of it comes from. Isn't it interesting that people have been made to feel anxiety toward the living food in their diets because of pesticides when the cooked, dead food is responsible for over 90 *percent* of the very chemicals with which they are concerned? I don't want to infer that you shouldn't be concerned—you should. The use of these deadly toxins on our food supply is a national disgrace. Wash everything as well as you can and purchase organically grown produce when available, and that is the best you can do. If you truly want to reduce the amount of pesticides in your diet, eat fewer animal products.

Dashing the hopes of a morning
with a cup of warm coffee.

—HENRY DAVID THOREAU

---

13. This last one is for you coffee drinkers. You know who you are. So many times someone will say to me, "I only have one cup of coffee a day in the morning. Is that so bad?" I will tell you that, ideally, you should not have coffee during the morning hours. Coffee is pure acid, and it does not, in any way, promote and support what we are trying to achieve here. Now, to reality. People who must have their one cup are going to do it, and in actual fact it's not going to disrupt the elimination cycle even close to the degree that cooked food will. After all, it is a liquid and will leave the stomach quickly. Sometimes it's just that the person wants something hot. Perhaps you could have a naturally caffeine-free herbal tea or hot water with lemon. Then again, there are some people who just happen to love the taste of coffee, and they just have to have that one cup. If this describes you, here's my recommendation: When you first wake up in the morning to start a new day, why make the very first thing you put into your living body something that is dead and acid-forming? Even if you have your one cup shortly thereafter, make the first thing to enter your body something alive. Celebrate the fact that God has

allowed you to awaken to the light of a new day with *life*. Have a glass of juice or a slice of melon or an orange. Wait ten to fifteen minutes and then have your coffee. Then have more fruit and fruit juice until noon. That's how to do it. There is a tremendous psychological benefit to consciously committing to have something living be the first thing to enter your body each day. It's a statement to the universe that you're for life. Isn't that exactly what we're shootin' for here—to be fit for life?

Whatever you do, don't put too much pressure on yourself with this. Start slowly if you have to. There's no rush. After you have done the one-week test and you are convinced that fruit 'til noon truly is the key to health that I have described, take it slow at first if you need to. What I mean by that is, some people can go straight to fruit only until noon with no problem. They have some ability to make such a dramatic change with ease. For others it doesn't come so easily. If it is something you don't feel you can do all at once, start by having fruit until noon every other day and make the transition a more gradual one. On those days that you don't eat fruit all the way until noon, at least make fruit and fruit juice the first thing you eat, and if you can only go to nine or ten or eleven o'clock, so be it. There is no right or wrong way here. As long as you are making an effort, it's right.

CHAPTER SIX

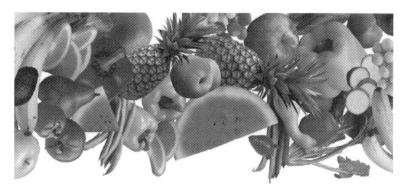

KEY TO SUCCESS #3:
LIFE IS IN THE BALANCE

Mere survival is an affliction.
What is of interest is life, and
the direction of that life.

—GUY FREGAULT

It seems that as time goes by, instead of the answer to successful weight loss becoming easier and easier, it becomes harder. It's more complicated, more involved, more difficult, more perplexing, more elusive. There is just so darn much to think about: all protein, no protein; high carbohydrate, low carbohydrate; how much fat; how much sugar; what about calories; portion measuring; meal replacements; fasting; dieting; drugs; surgery; what's my blood type; what's my body type; what's my emotional type? This dizzying array of factors, and more, is what people are confronted with when the subject of weight loss comes up. Why? How on God's good Earth has something as normal and natural and necessary to life as *eating* become such an uphill task, such a chore? My friends, it's time to simplify, before all hope is lost.

Every one of the factors listed above is irrelevant. There is no need to think of any of them. Your success comes down to the *one* factor this book is based upon: Eat more living food than cooked food. Free your mind. Wouldn't you prefer to focus your efforts on one factor instead of more than a dozen?

The first Key to Success is the importance of dividing the food you eat into 50 percent living food and 50 percent cooked food. The second Key to Success is instrumental in reaching that goal. In addition to the numerous life-enhancing benefits of eating fruit 'til noon, doing so raises the amount of living food to about one-third of your overall food intake. That's a huge step, especially if you were at 10 percent or less of living food. The way to reach the ultimate goal of 50 percent—50 percent will obviously be determined by what is eaten at the other two primary meals of the day, lunch and dinner. And once again, it is simplicity personified. No complicated instructions to follow, no convoluted procedures to undertake, even though you may not understand the reasoning behind them. No deprivation that leaves you hungry and wanting at the end of a meal. No powdered drinks instead of food. You get to eat. I'm not saying it won't be different from what you're accustomed to, because without doing something different, where are we? Changes in habits *must* be made for there to be a change in conditions. What you will find is that what I'm going to propose will be understandable, sensible, logical and doable.

Here is the challenge before us: to incorporate enough living food—that is fruits and vegetables—in the diet so that it comprises at least half of what is eaten in total. There are three primary meals of the day: breakfast, lunch and dinner. Breakfast is already taken of: It's fruit 'til noon, which I just pointed out is a giant step in reaching your goal of 50 percent living food. Obviously, that leaves lunch and dinner to supply the remaining living food. Since the fruit eaten throughout the morning will supply about 25 percent of the 50 percent needed to fulfill the goal, the other approximately 25 percent needs to come from lunch and dinner. And that means *salads*. I don't mean a scrap of lettuce with a cherry tomato pushed over to the side of a plate loaded down with cooked food, nor am I talking about some meager, token salad on a little plate the size of a teacup saucer. I'm talking about a full-on, righteous-sized salad with lots of ingredients. After all, this will be the *living* part of the meal. That's not where to skimp. Lettuce, of which there are many varieties, as well as tomato, cucumber, spinach, sprouts, celery, carrots, bell peppers—you know—a *salad*, in its own bowl or on its own plate, in order to give it the stature it deserves.

> **O**ne hath no better thing
> under the sun than to eat and to
> drink and to be merry.
>
> —ECCLESIASTES 8:14

I have come up with a simple formula. Following it will enable you to eat, and eat well and plenty of, the foods you enjoy and don't want to give up, plus it will amply supply the living food required to make all this work. Aside from fruits and vegetables, the two primary types of food to eat are referred to as the concentrated foods: proteins and starches. Proteins are all meat, chicken, fish, eggs, dairy and soy products. Starches are potatoes, pasta, bread and all grains, such as rice, barley, oats, millet, couscous, etc. Here it is as simply as I can possibly put it so there can be no con-fusion: For lunch, have one or the other concentrated foods, either a protein or a starch, and along with it have vegetables and a salad. For dinner, it's the same thing: a protein or a starch with vegetables and a salad. That's it.

Before I give you some specific examples to make sure you are clear about what I'm suggesting, let me clarify something about having vegetables and salad. Right now you might correctly be thinking, "Vegetables and salads are the same thing; salads *are* vegetables." Right you are. But for the sake of what I'm presenting here, I have to make a distinction between the two. When I talk about having vegetables with a salad, I'm talking about having *cooked* vegetables. A salad, in this book, will always be referring to a raw salad of mixed greens and the like. True, some people like to eat raw vegetables that are traditionally cooked such as cauliflower, broccoli, green beans and others, and they most certainly are living, as is a salad. But when I say to have a protein, vegetables and a salad, or a starch, vegetables and a salad, the vegetables are prepared in some way. Either steamed, sautéed, grilled, baked or otherwise prepared with heat.

The second question that immediately arises as regards eating prepared vegetables is, "Do I count them as cooked food or living food?" The answer is neither. They're neutral. It should go without saying that vegetables shouldn't be overcooked until they're nothing but mush. When you lightly steam or sauté vegetables, yes, they are cooked somewhat, but they still have value. Their fiber content is still available, as well as some nutrients. Say, for example, you want to have a steak. Have it with a salad and some well-prepared vegetables. If, on the other hand, you are craving pasta, have *it* with a salad and vegetables. You want broiled chicken or fish? Have either one with salad and vegetables. Rice and vegetables? Have it with a salad. Maybe you don't want either a protein or a starch, and you only want vegetables and a salad. Great! Whatever you have for lunch, have it with a salad, and whatever you have for dinner, have it with a salad.

What if one day you are craving both a steak *and* pasta? Have one for lunch with salad and vegetables, and have the other for dinner with salad and vegetables. This way you can have whatever you want, just not all at the same meal. Of course, on occasion you will have both a protein and a starch together, such as a sandwich, a hamburger, lasagna or pizza, but for the most part, on most occasions, you would be well served to have one or the other, not both together. The reason that I'm suggesting you don't have a protein and a starch at the same meal has to do with energy.

We already know that digestion requires more energy than anything else, and there is only a certain amount available each day to carry out all the processes of life, including the elimination of waste, which is crucial in weight loss. So anything that can be done to streamline digestion (or to lighten the load of the digestive process, which in turn conserves energy) would certainly make good sense, don't you think? It is obvious that some foods require more energy for digestion than others. We know that fruit requires none, but everything else does in varying degrees. The concentrated foods—proteins and starches—require considerably more energy to be broken down than do the plant foods, vegetables and salads. One of the primary reasons that this approach to weight loss works so well is its judicious, intelligent use of available energy.

To squander energy unnecessarily when it can be not only conserved, but actually put to better use elsewhere, only serves to sabotage your efforts. It's not as though there is an inexhaustible supply on hand each day. This may be an oversimplistic way of putting it, but the energy you force to be used on digesting a second concentrated food at any given meal is energy that could have been used by the body in its efforts to lose weight. Simplistic though it may be, it's accurate. The amount of energy you have on hand each day can be likened to having a certain amount of money to put toward debts. If you have four ongoing debts you are paying off and $1,000 to put toward them, you can either pay $250 toward each of the four or put it all toward only three. In that case, the fourth receives nothing. Think of lunch and dinner every day for a month. That's sixty meals. If at each one of those meals only one concentrated food (either a protein or a starch) required digestive energy, can you see the advantage of that over *two* concentrated foods (both a protein and a starch) using up energy at all those meals?

Besides, concentrated foods are heavier and more filling. At a meal with two concentrated foods (both a protein and a starch), you are more likely to finish them and *not* have enough room for the salad. Big mistake. Conserving energy from the digestive process is an extremely wise and beneficial thing to do, and giving the digestive system less work to do accomplishes that task. Over time the benefits of doing so are revealed.

There is another basis for not mixing proteins and starches at the same meal. It's called proper food combining. If you are familiar with the original *Fit for Life*, you know that a good portion of that book advocated the proper combination of proteins and starches. If you recall, I already mentioned that from age three to twenty-five I had the most debilitating and painful stomach disorder. It filled my youth with pain and drugs to quell the pain. I loved to eat, but every time I did my body was wracked with pain. It was the bane of my existence, plain and simple. At age twenty-five, in 1970, I started to combine proteins and starches properly, and as if by magic not only did I immediately stop having stomach and digestive disorders, but to this day, I have not experienced the least bit of discomfort or pain after meals. One of the main reasons that I wanted to write *Fit for Life* was to share the good news about proper food combining, which has been a subject of study and numerous books for at least three-quarters of a century.

> The vast majority of human beings dislike and even actually dread all notions with which they are not familiar. . . .
> Hence it comes about that at their first appearance innovators have always been derided as fools and madmen.
>
> —ALDOUS HUXLEY

Proper food combining has also been a subject of con-
troversy—not amongst those who have had experiences
such as mine and found relief from stomach and digestive
pain after years of suffering, but from the same group of
people who are convinced that you can cook all the life out
of food and still receive the same benefit from it that you
would from food that is still living. I can assure you that the
numerous people who have discovered the benefits of properly combining foods laugh out loud at the "experts" who
insist that it doesn't work.

It is not my intent to defend proper food combining or
even go into it at great length. I only want to touch on it
briefly as it is relevant to the subject at hand. It is simply
this: Proteins require an acid digestive juice, and starches
require an alkaline digestive juice. Remember Chemistry
101? Mix an acid and an alkaline together, and they are
neutralized. When digestive juices are neutralized in the
stomach, the entire digestive process is prolonged, wasting
the precious energy you are trying to conserve. The food
spoils, creates pain and sends millions of people running to
the medicine cabinet for relief. Sound familiar?

The fact is that not everyone experiences acid indigestion, gas or heartburn when they eat proteins and starches
together, and to be perfectly honest with you, I can't
explain why. But there are many people who stop experiencing these discomforts when they don't eat proteins and
starches at the same meal. And that's a fact. Fortunately, it
proves itself as quickly and as definitively as eating only
fruit 'til noon. If you try it and it works for you, then what
more evidence do you need?

You don't have to concern yourself with any of the particulars of proper food combining. I have told you throughout that if you commit to eating at least 50 percent living food, that is all you will have to focus on to be successful. My reason for asking you to have *either* a protein or a starch at meals with vegetables and salad, and not *both* at the same meal, has to do with energy conservation. One type of concentrated food requires less energy for digestion than two concentrated foods, and that's the long and short of it. I don't want to become annoying by harping on the same thing, but any time you can use less energy to digest a meal you are, in effect, putting money in the bank—energy not used for digestion is available to the body for use in cleansing and healing, elimination and weight loss.

When I said that the subject of mixing foods has been discussed for at least three-quarters of a century, that's in the modern era. There are references to it going back centuries. Remember the passage I quoted on not cooking food from the *Essene Gospel of Peace,* which was supposedly attributed to Jesus? Well, in the same passage he discussed the mixing of different types of food when he said, "Cook not, neither mix all things all with another, lest your bowels become like steaming bogs. For I tell you truly if you mix together all sorts of food in your body, then the peace of your body will cease, and endless war will rage in you."[1] Steaming bogs—that's some fairly descriptive language, wouldn't you say?

Once again, just as I did with the last Key to Success on eating fruit 'til noon, I'm going to end this chapter with an overview and some tips on how to be most successful.

Tips and Hints for Balancing Your Meals with Living Food

1. The greatest tip I can give you is to encourage you to fix in your mind the never-ending need your living body has for living food. How well your body functions, how effectively it transforms food into energy, how capable it is of absorbing nutrients, and how efficiently it removes wastes—all depend upon how much living food the body has to work with. Having this awareness in your consciousness can only help you. I'm not suggesting that it become an all-consuming preoccupation that you fixate on until it becomes a chore. If you merely acknowledge that it is a priority in your life on a subtle level, your higher self will instinctively and automatically direct you to do what will be in the living body's best interest. When your mentality is that a meal is not complete without a fair share of living food, salads will start to take on the importance they deserve.

   When you drive in your car, you know to fasten your seatbelt. Once in a while, you will fail to put your seatbelt on, but you know it's the wise and intelligent thing to do. The same can be said for making living food a priority at your meals. It becomes a way of life.

The unfortunate thing about this world is
that good habits are so much easier
to give up than bad ones.

—W. SOMERSET MAUGHAM

---

2. Let's talk about salads. Have you ever heard people say, on being asked if they would like a salad, "Oh, no thanks, I already had a salad today." You never hear someone say, "Oh, no thanks, I already had meat today." People will have bacon or sausage in the morning, then roast beef or a hamburger or chicken for lunch, and then when dinner comes around and they are offered a steak, you don't ever hear it turned down because they already had meat earlier in the day. But people will have a salad at lunch, and that precludes them from having one at dinner. Why is that?

How in the world has it come to be that the one part of the meal that is the most important for health, the living part, is the one that can't be repeated at another meal? It's almost as though the mind-set is one of getting it (salad) out of the way so full attention can be put toward the cooked, lifeless food. I don't know exactly what psychological conditioning has brought this about, but I do know that it has not benefited us and needs to be changed.

3. Some people prefer to have salad by itself; others prefer to eat it with the meal. I have been asked if it's

healthier to eat it before, during or after the meal. As far as the benefits are concerned, it makes no difference. If I had to choose when to best have it I would say either before or with the meal, preferably before, but *not* after. The reasoning for this should be fairly obvious. Have it first and you have fulfilled the living food part of the meal. Then you can have the cooked part of the meal. This way, if you become full before finishing, at least you know you have had the part of the meal that will best fuel your body. On the other hand, if you hold off having your salad until the end of the meal, by the time you get to it you may either be too full to finish it, or you might eat it even though you're full, thereby overeating, which is equally detrimental.

4. One of the reasons that salads have been treated like the "unwanted stepchild" and eaten with the attitude of "getting it out of the way" is that so little attention has been put into them that they are usually boring and unimaginative. That is tragic, considering that there is a seemingly infinite number of variations for innovative and delectable salads.

    I want to introduce you to a concept for eating salads that may very well revolutionize the way you eat. It certainly will do so if your attitude toward salad is a wedge of lettuce with a glop of mayonnaise as dressing. This concept was first originated by my ex-wife, Marilyn, back in the early 1980s.

    Although Marilyn and I are no longer married, we are still close, and for seventeen years I was the lucky recipient of her culinary artistry, ingenuity and mastery. There's no other way to say it: She is a genius in the kitchen. She has that certain "something," a magical touch that can turn the most mundane ingredients into a feast fit for royalty. Many times she would go into the kitchen to prepare something and say, "There's really not too much to work with here, but I'll come up with something." Then she would come out with some spectacularly delectable banquet that would have everyone swooning with delight. It was a running joke around our house to see how long it would take dinner guests to start hinting around as to when they might once again be invited over for one of "Mare's spreads."

The concept she came up with, which has now been copied far and wide, is the Main Course Salad, a term she coined for the original *Fit for Life* book. Main Course Salads are, in a word, a godsend for this approach to eating. They are convenient, fun, delicious and satisfying, and they support completely the goal of living food comprising half your overall diet. The principle of having a concentrated food (either protein or starch) with vegetables and salad is still adhered to, only not in the traditional way of a separate bowl or plate of salad next to another plate with your chicken or fish or pasta or rice, with vegetables on the side. Instead, the Main Course Salad combines everything in one nourishing, gustatory sensation.

Main Course Salads are easy to make, and with a little ingenuity, the possible variations are practically endless. They work for either lunch or dinner. If you get into making these, I'm telling you, they will become an integral part of your diet. A week never passes that I don't have several.

I can easily think of at least six that are my very favorites, but I'm going to tell you of two so you can have an idea of what I'm talking about. Remember, the variations are limited only by your imagination. The ingredients I'm going to mention can be changed or substituted with absolutely anything you desire. Apart from adhering to the basic principle of a protein or starch with vegetables mixed into a salad, there is no right or wrong, no rules, no limitations—it's whatever you are partial to.

I love potatoes. There must be two hundred ways of serving potatoes, and I love 'em all. I'm also one of those people who can't get enough broccoli. I know there are many people who can't stand it, but well-prepared and seasoned-just-right broccoli is one of the most versatile and tasty vegetables there is. The character Newman on *Seinfeld* would disagree. Jerry once said to him, "You wouldn't eat broccoli if it was deep fried in chocolate sauce." Newman, to prove him wrong, took a bite and immediately spit it out, exclaiming, "Vile weed!"

> **W**eed—a plant whose virtues have
> not yet been discovered.
>
> —RALPH WALDO EMERSON

First, lightly steam chunks of potato (any type) about a half-inch or so in size along with broccoli florets. Then sauté the potato and broccoli in a pan with a little butter or olive oil, add garlic or minced onion, salt and pepper, or whatever spices you like, and let them cool down while you prepare a big salad with lettuce (one type or several), spinach, cucumber, tomatoes, red cabbage—whatever ingredients you like. Mix it all together, add a dressing of your liking and dive in. My mouth is watering just writing about it. For those of you Newman types who would rather eat lawn clippings than broccoli, you can substitute any vegetable or vegetables you prefer: peas and corn, zucchini, asparagus, green beans, whatever.

The same can be done with a protein of your choice. Say you want steak. You can use filet, strip, rib-eye, whichever you want. Prepare it in strips sautéed, broiled or grilled. Same with chunks of chicken or shrimp. Prepare the vegetables you want, mix it all together with your salad, add the dressing and there it is.

Main Course Salads are complete meals that not only taste fantastic, satisfy your desire to eat and allow the eating experience to remain a pleasurable one, they also nourish the body with the living food it needs to function at its highest level. And you can create so many variations on the theme. It is as though they were created for the expressed purpose of encouraging and simplifying this approach to eating. If you want ideas for dozens of different Main Course Salads (and regular salads), you can thumb through the original *Fit for Life*, *Fit for Life II* or *The American Vegetarian Cookbook from the Fit for Life Kitchen*. You'll have more than enough ideas to last a lifetime—a healthy and fit lifetime.

5. It's an understatement to say that the dressing is an important part of any salad. In fact, it is the one ingredient you can least do without. Who wants a salad without dressing? Bugs Bunny maybe. Let me be crystal-clear on this. You should have absolutely any salad dressing in order to more fully enjoy your salads. If the worst thing you ever do dietetically is use a slightly inferior salad dressing, prepare now to figure out what you want to do on your one-hundredth birthday. Having said that, allow me to qualify it a bit. If you want to use store-bought dressings, there's no problem with that. There are two kinds of dressing, however. There is the kind that adds MSG, nitrates, food coloring, artificial flavors and all manner of other multisyllablic chemicals that are designed to make your liver and kidneys work overtime. And there is the kind that uses good, pure ingredients and no chemical additives. Want to venture a guess as to which one I would recommend?

Health-food stores have a dizzying array of high-quality, totally delicious salad dressings. You don't have to give up any of the flavor you're looking for, only the chemical ingredients. Seek them out— you're worth it. A great brand that has many different varieties of delicious dressings, without a bunch of chemical additives, is Newman's Own. Not only are these dressings tasty and devoid of all the chemicals that are to be avoided, but all profits from the sale of Paul Newman's products are donated to charitable organizations.

Remember that most dressings (unless specifically made with low-fat ingredients) generally contain seven to ten grams of fat per tablespoon. Knowing this, keep in mind that you can easily turn what would be a healthy meal into an unncessarily high-fat one by being too heavy-handed with the dressing.

You can make your own dressings as well, if you like. You would start with a high-quality olive oil, add lemon or lime juice, salt, seasoned salt or salt-free seasonings. To that basic dressing, which is delicious on its own, you can add various ingredients: either some mayonnaise to turn it into a creamy dressing, Dijon mustard, barbecue sauce, honey or anything else you want, along with ground pepper, garlic or any kind of herb or spice you are partial to. Most important of all, you should truly love the dressing so that you look forward to your salads with relish. Oh, that reminds me, you could add relish to your dressings also. To make it easier to use your own healthy, homemade dressings, you can make a large amount of dressing at the beginning of the week and put it in a bottle to have each day with your salads rather than having to prepare a dressing for each individual salad or always being forced to use a store-bought dressing to save time.

6. I hope you have fully grasped the importance of easing the workload of the digestive system and the benefits that can be realized by doing so. We know that the digestive system has to deal with some seventy tons of food in a lifetime, and the energy used to accomplish that impressive feat is more than all other expenditures of energy combined. Therefore, any action you can take (however large or small) that results in less energy being used for digestion automatically increases your chances of success in direct proportion to the amount of energy saved. In this regard, we humans are energy-producing eating machines. The more we eat and the more complex the food we eat, the more energy is used up. The less we eat and the less complex the food we eat, the more energy we have for other bodily functions. As the realization of this physiological truth becomes more and more real to you, this entire approach to eating will take on a much deeper meaning.

In describing the third Key to Success, that of balancing the amount of living food with cooked food, I spoke of the importance of having only one type of concentrated food, either a protein or a starch, with vegetables and salad. Obviously, the reason for doing so is to use less energy during the digestive process. As you start to eat this way, you will undoubtedly wonder at some point if it is less objectionable to eat a protein with another protein or a starch with another starch than it is to eat a protein with a starch. Even though two proteins or two starches together are two concentrated foods, at least they are of the same type so, yes, if you are having protein at a meal you can have more than one, and same for two starches.

As an example, if you are going to have steak or fish or chicken along with your vegetables and salad, you may want to have a shrimp cocktail as an appetizer. That's fine. Or even surf 'n' turf, which is lobster and steak, both proteins. On the starch side, perhaps you're having pasta primavera, which is pasta prepared with a tasty sauce and an array of vegetables. That and your salad is the meal. If you're like me, you like garlic bread with pasta, and since bread and pasta both are starches, that's fine also. But I have to caution you. If you are going to have two proteins or two starches at the same meal, it *must not* be at the expense of your salad. Eat your salad first if need be; that way, you're sure to get the living part of the meal. Then eat the other foods until you are satisfied. This way, when you're full and leaving something unfinished, it's the cooked part, not the living part.

Never cease to be convinced
that life might be better.

—ANDRÉ GIDE

---

7. Dining out. For some reason, people hear this new
   approach to eating and frequently ask, "Well, what
   about eating out? Can I still do this?" Why not? First
   of all, sometimes you're going to dine out and eat
   whatever you darn well please. Proteins and starches
   mixed together, no salad, and fruit for dessert. That's
   just how life is. But based on your level of commitment to eat well *and* lose weight, eating like that is
   going to comprise but a small percentage of your
   meals. Overall, it is a simple matter to eat out and
   still be in alignment with what you have learned
   here. All you do is decide before the meal if you are
   having proteins or starches, then plan your meal
   around that decision.

   Let's say you're in the mood for a steak. Once
   you've decided that, your main hurdle will be getting
   past what I refer to as the "commitment tester,"
   which is always brought to the table before you've
   even seen the menu: the basket of bread. Bread is a
   starch. It's concentrated and is not ideal with the
   steak, which is a concentrated protein. Instead, you
   can have an appetizer that is either vegetable or protein: crab-stuffed mushrooms, shrimp cocktail or a
   bowl of soup without starch. Then your steak with
   vegetables (not a potato) and your salad. That's a

good meal. Plenty of food and you won't be over-burdening the digestive process, which squanders energy and leaves you feeling "heavy." Take note of how much lighter you will feel after this meal than in the past when you've eaten it with potatoes and bread.

As regards not having the traditional potato with the steak, I know it tastes good, but it's simply too much. It's too heavy to have two different concentrated foods at once like that. Potatoes have for so long been served as an accompaniment to some protein dish that it's strange to think of them as an entrée. But I will tell you a baked potato with butter and a salad with some tastily prepared vegetables is a wonderfully healthy, delicious meal. And ordering a steak and asking for the vegetable of the day along with it instead of the potato is not going to make you a village outcast who is forever shunned.

Remember those old-time westerns where a bunch of cowboys are sitting around a table playing poker and all of the sudden one of them jumps up, pushing his chair over with the back of his knees when he stands, and says, "Hey mister, you're cheatin' and I'm callin' you out"? Well, no one is going to jump up like that when you forgo the potato with the steak and say, "Hey, what's goin' on here, you in some kinda cult or something?" As a matter of fact, I have noticed that people are genuinely interested and curious as to why a special point is made of not having the potato. And that gives you the opportunity to share the life-enhancing information you have learned, thereby performing a service for your fellow diner. And I will tell you from experience that the gratitude displayed by those who sincerely appreciate your sharing something that can help them feel better is a lot more satisfying than dessert. Which, if it were fruit, you would already have eaten *before* the meal.

If you decide to go with starches, you can then welcome the "commitment tester." Follow it with pasta, vegetables and salad. No protein foods at that meal. You always get to eat what you like and be satisfied—you just don't have everything you like at every meal.

It is a simple, intelligent, common-sense approach to eating that becomes second nature the more it is practiced. And these small alterations in your eating habits that result in more living food and less work for the digestive process, which frees up energy, are a very small price to pay for being able to enjoy the eating experience and lose weight in the process.

8. There is a habit many people have at meals that appears on the surface to be harmless enough but, in fact, is not such a good idea: drinking water or other liquids with food. There's a perfectly reasonable explanation. I have made the case, almost to the point of being annoying, that all steps that can be made to streamline (rather than hinder) the digestive process should be taken. Digestive juices are liquid. When liquid enters the stomach it dilutes those digestive juices and washes some from the stomach, forcing the

body to use up energy by secreting more. I have seen people guzzle glass after glass of water during the course of a meal. Frequently when they feel overly full, bloated and gassy after the meal, they don't attribute it to the fact that they kept diluting the digestive juices and washing them from the stomach.

If you wish to have water with your meals, there is a more sensible way to do so. Take very small sips throughout the meal, just enough to wash your palate. That's all you have to do, and you won't retard the digestive process. A particularly healthy habit to cultivate is to drink a full glass of water immediately prior to eating a meal. I think you will find that you won't be nearly as thirsty during the meal when you drink a glass of water beforehand.

> It's a naive wine without any breeding,
> but I think you'll be amused
> by its presumption.
>
> —JAMES THURBER

I can feel the wine enthusiasts holding their breath, waiting to see where "the grape" fits into the scheme of things. Okay, you can exhale. I like wine, especially when eating out. It always seems to make a meal more festive and relaxing. The way I drink wine is to have a glass before the meal, then sip it the same way I would if it were water: very small sips so as not to flood the stomach. See? There's a way to have everything you want.

9. There are, generally speaking, two times a day when people like to snack, between lunch and dinner, and in the evening. I didn't mention between breakfast and lunch because if you're having fruit until noon, that means you can have fruit right up until about thirty minutes before lunch. Snacks seem innocent enough, but they have the potential of either supporting and furthering your health goals, or pulling the reins in on them.

The most useful advice I can give you is to, as best you can, eat something living for a snack. There will, in all likelihood, be times when you have a candy bar or chips or cookies, or some other such thing, and it's not the end of the world, but if you can satisfy your desire for something to nibble on between meals with a living food you will be doing yourself a great service. And by now you certainly know why. In addition to helping increase your balance of living food over cooked food and supplying your body with the nutrients it needs to perform the functions of life, their digestion is energy-efficient. Snacks that are living have their enzymes intact. That means very little effort is required for digestion because that's what the enzymes in the food do. Once the enzymes have been destroyed, the body has to manufacture its own digestive enzymes, which use up the precious enzymes that could have been used for cleansing and weight loss.

When you do want to have a snack that is living, I recommend you choose from three: vegetables, fruits, or nuts and seeds. It has almost become a cliché to suggest snacking on carrot and/or celery sticks. But the fact is, they are highly nutritious, energy-efficient and they are alkaline foods, which help neutralize acid in the body, a most beneficial bonus.

Fruits make a great snack, especially raisins, dates and dried fruit. They're easy to carry around, stay in the stomach a bit longer to keep you from feeling hungry and are available in the bloodstream as energy within an hour. That is a gigantic plus when you are seeking an afternoon lift without having to resort to caffeine or sugar.

Nuts and seeds are also a very convenient and beneficial snack, but there are some guidelines to follow when eating them. First and most important, they must be raw, not roasted. Raw, they are alkaline; roasted, they are totally acid, plus their enzymes are destroyed. Because nuts are a concentrated food, they should not be overeaten, which is easy to do if you're not careful. One good-sized handful should be all you have at one time. I'm partial to raw almonds and cashews, and pumpkin and sunflower seeds. I find that people generally want to snack on something around four in the afternoon. A handful of nuts or seeds at that time will easily hold off your hunger until dinner. Here's a tip: For years, whenever I have nuts as a snack, which I do two or three times a week, I like to have cucumber with them. If you haven't had this it may sound strange, but it is delicious and the cucumber seems to help move the nuts through the system more efficiently. I peel the cucumbers and cut them into spears or rounds, and they always taste great and hold off my hunger for hours. Just try it once, and you'll see what I mean.

In England, there is a wonderful tradition known as high tea. At four in the afternoon, which is a few hours after lunch and a few hours before dinner, a light snack is eaten with tea. It's usually "mini" sandwiches or pastries, and it's done in a ceremonial fashion with fancy silver and china. Seems like 4:00 P.M. is the universal time when people need something. I bring this up because there are times when people who are striving diligently to lose weight still have a craving every so often for something sweet other than fruit. Chocolate. A piece of cake or pie. Or candy. Since having these types of sweets as a dessert is truly detrimental, the best time to have them is when the stomach is empty. In other words, around 4:00 P.M.—high tea. That way you know your stomach is empty, and you won't be eating for several more hours. That's the healthier way to have sweets.

If I'd known I was gonna live this long,
I'd have taken better care of myself.

—EUBIE BLAKE

---

10. This last tip is one I have found to be immensely beneficial for overall health and instrumental in helping the body shed weight. It's not something that is a must, but it definitely accelerates your success and supports all your efforts in a big way. One day a week, have a totally living day—nothing cooked for twenty-four hours. You have fruit and juice, smoothies, vegetables and their juices, and raw salads. People are different, I know. Some can start to have one living day a week with no problem. Others find it more difficult and have to build up to it. Just make the effort, and it will quickly become apparent what a good thing it is on all levels. After eating cooked food every day of your life, to suddenly give the body a complete rest from having to deal with cooked food is a major boon.

I have noticed among people who make this effort a pronounced increase in their feelings of accomplishment that spurs them on to even greater resolve. You feel wonderful after a day of only living food. You truly get a feel for the power and ability you have to effect a positive change in your life.

Perhaps you can build up to having only living food one day a week by first trying one day a week where you have only fruit until your evening meal, or only fruit and salad until your evening meal. So you are only having one cooked meal that day. Any way you want to do it, it all works in your favor. There are lots of ways of using living food to your benefit, and the longer you incorporate this way of eating into your lifestyle, the more the possibilities will reveal themselves to you. The important thing is that you start, and let your body begin to reap the benefits that automatically result from increasing the amount of living food you eat. The fact is, as you will find out, there are going to be days where you simply won't feel like eating anything heavy. You just won't feel like it. It's something your body dictates. You may wake up one morning and only want to have fruit and juice the entire day. It is important that you are sensitive to these feelings and inclinations and know that *any* time you substitute a cooked meal with a living one, you are enhancing your overall health and increasing your chances for successful weight loss.

On a personal note, I can tell you that I go for long periods of time when I eat only living food every other day. At some point down the road, it may be something you want to try. If the concept of eating more living food is new to you, the idea of eating *only* living food every other day may very well be as appealing as sticking your finger in an electrical socket. I know how daunting an idea it can be. And I'm not saying it's something you have to do to be successful; it's not. It took me years to get to the place of being able to do it for long periods of time. But if you want to superaccelerate your progress, or just want to see how really great you can feel, that's how to do it. On the days you eat cooked food, you follow the recommendations already given: fruit and fruit juices until noon, then lunch of a concentrated food (either a protein or a starch) with vegetables and salad, and dinner of a different concentrated food with vegetables and salad.

Better bend than break.

—Scottish Proverb

Before moving on, I wish to revisit the subject of using this information in a relaxed atmosphere of flexibility. This needs to be a very fluid, easily adaptable way of eating in order for it to be a lifestyle. If it is turned into a forced march where every little supposed transgression is met with guilt and rigidity, it won't work. For some reason, when it comes to dietary changes, many people become very unforgiving taskmasters and lay a lot of guilt on themselves. It only leads to frustration. Nothing is carved in granite here. There will be times when you eat a big breakfast or drink pasteurized juice. There will be meals that have more cooked food than living food or meals with proteins and starches mixed together. There will be times when you don't eat a salad with your meal, or you will eat cooked food all day with no fruit or salad at all. There will be times like that. Maybe at a party or on vacation or when what you want is simply not available, you will have what's convenient even though it is not exactly in line with the principles you are endeavoring to follow. That's life! If you can keep the big picture in mind and concentrate on the direction you are taking in your life and not get hung up on the intricate specifics of every last meal, you will be a much happier, healthier person on all levels—physically, emotionally and spiritually. It is far more important to be able to look back over your life at the end of the year and be pleased with what you did overall than to scrutinize every meal of every day. Be flexible. Make it fun. Be kind and forgiving to yourself—and, most importantly, be congratulatory for the efforts you have made and the accomplishments you have achieved. That's what being fit for life is all about.

CHAPTER SEVEN

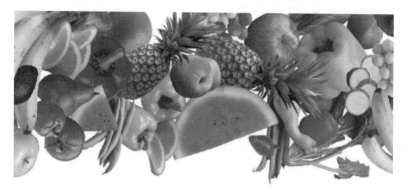

BENEFITS AND REWARDS

The poorest would not part
with health for money, but the richest
would gladly part with all their
money for health.

—C. C. COLTON

Considering the title and contents of this book, I think it would be safe to say that you have at least *some* interest in losing weight. If you have been trying for a long time, it is also likely that you have had to endure the disappointments of past attempts that ended in frustration, despite all the promises and assurances of how "fast and easy" it would be to drop the weight. If that is the case, you must be hoping beyond hope that this does not fall into the category of what the Federal Trade Commission recently said 55 percent of all weight-loss ads are: "Blatantly misleading or outright lies."[1]

Since I myself have, in the past, succumbed to the hype only to be disappointed in the end, I have made a point of refraining from making over-the-top promises that your success is guaranteed with little or no effort. Because of my own success with eating a diet predominated by living food, or at least 50 percent living food, and the success of numerous other people over the years, I am confident that if you will commit to doing what you have learned here, you will enjoy gradual but steady weight loss until you are at the weight you wish to be.

I would further venture to say that, if you do indeed lose the weight you want to lose, you probably wouldn't mind simultaneously experiencing an improvement in your health overall. That's a little like asking if you wouldn't mind having a free car to go along with your lottery winnings.

In an earlier chapter, I made the point that weight loss and improved health go hand-in-hand. They are, in fact, inseparable. You can't have a coin with only one side. And the flip side of the weight-loss coin is an improvement in health. You really can't have one without the other. When the body is in a state of good health, it is best able to shed weight. It is a misnomer to suggest that you can be over-weight *and* in good health. Overweight is *not* a feature of good health. When in good health the body automatically normalizes its weight. Being overweight is a statement that your body is not as healthy as it could be. What you will never hear from the dreaded 55 percent of weight-loss ads that hedge the truth to make a sale is that weight loss does not happen in a vacuum. It happens when the necessary conditions for weight loss are in place.

> Health is the first and greatest
> of all blessings.
>
> —LORD CHESTERFIELD

Throughout this book, I have been praising the supreme, unsurpassed intelligence that resides in the human body. Once this exquisite machine is animated by the breath of life, it automatically strives for the very highest level of health possible. It can do nothing else as this striving is hardwired into its very cell structure. The reason you are able to lose weight with this particular approach is *because* you are healthier. By properly fueling the body with more living food, all systems function at a higher level. This enables the body to more readily lose weight, which in turn increases overall well-being. As your health *increases,* your weight *decreases.* It is a synergistic undertaking that the living body initiates on its own behalf. So, in addition to the weight you will be losing, I want to go over a few of the other positive results you can look forward to as a consequence of properly fueling your body with living food.

1. **And the First Prize Is . . .** On the physical level of life, what do you think would be the most prized gift of all? Even though your first guess might be more money than could possibly be spent in a lifetime, what good is all that money if the possessor is too sick to enjoy it? If a magic genie were to offer you one or the other, health or wealth, what would you choose? If you *knew* you could live out your life free of pain, ill health and disease and could experience a consistent, high-energy, vital life of well-being, is there *anything* you would choose over that?

> The whole world is a series of balanced antagonisms.
>
> —RALPH WALDO EMERSON

Do you think it's possible to live life like that *without* a magic genie? Don't you think that the intelligence that governs all life—God—would provide at least the possibility of such a life, or have you been convinced that as time goes by something has to hurt or break down? Isn't life full of opposites? Earlier I said that whatever belief a person holds, there is someone, somewhere, with the opposite belief. Opposites exist everywhere: life and death; positive and negative; good and bad; up and down; in and out; black and white; and, of course, health and ill health. It seems reasonable to suggest that if ill health exists, and it is rather apparent that it does, then health must exist also. I once read a review in a medical book that started with the following sentence: "From the perspective of the medical profession, healthy people are simply patients pausing briefly on their journey from disease to disease."[2] I'm not talking about fleeting intervals of health that are all too short and regularly overwhelmed by periods of ill health. No, I mean long-term, uninterrupted health.

Look at the astonishing human body that I have taken every opportunity to praise. No matter how eloquently and elegantly I attempt to describe the unsurpassed magnificence of the human body, I always feel as though I fall short of depicting its true splendor. There aren't sufficient words in the English language to do it justice. All who study the life sciences are humbled by the human body's awe-inspiring ability to perform feats of unimaginable complexity.

Is it at all possible that such a marvel of creation would be left without the power and means to protect itself and provide itself with a consistently, high level of health? Browse through any book on physiology and you are bound to be impressed. There are systems in place to oversee every last organ, activity and function of the body: the cardiovascular system (heart and blood), digestive system, muscular system, skeletal system, endocrine system (glands and hormones), nervous system (brain and spinal cord), integumentary system (skin, hair and nails), respiratory system, urinary system and reproductive system.

In determining whether any living organism is indeed living, five basic requisites must be met. It must be able to take in nutrition, perform the process of metabolism, be able to move on its own, reproduce and remove wastes. The human body meets all five. That last one, being able to remove wastes, warrants special mention. That is because any living organism that takes in food *must* be able to remove the wastes that are the automatic, spontaneous result of metabolism. If for any reason the ability to remove wastes is hindered, or worse yet, curtailed altogether, the organism would quickly die, poisoned by its own uneliminated wastes.

In constructing the incredible human machine, you can be certain beyond any possible doubt that the infinitely intelligent Grand Creator of all and everything did not forget to equip the human body with something as necessary as a mechanism to remove wastes. That would be like building a multibillion-dollar aircraft and forgetting to attach wings.

In the same way that the ten other systems of the body have their specific jobs and functions to perform, so it is with the system in charge of waste removal. It's called the lymphatic system (lymph system for short). The lymph system is, in fact, commonly referred to as the body's "garbage collector."

The lymph system is an astounding network of glands, nodes, nodules, vessels and fluid that totally permeates the interior of the body. There are some nodes the size of a nickel and some so small you can't see them with the naked eye. There are millions upon millions of them in numbers too great to count. We know that we are kept alive by the river of life, the bloodstream, that flows through some 90,000 miles of blood vessels. And as revealed earlier, there is *three times* as much lymph fluid in your body as there is blood. There literally isn't a spot the size of a pinpoint anywhere inside the body that does not come into direct contact with the lymph system. That is how exceedingly important it is for wastes to be gathered up from every last one of the 100 trillion cells, broken down and eliminated as quickly and efficiently as possible.

Here's an irony for you that borders on the bizarre. Most people, if not *all*, would like to live completely free of pain, ill health or disease. I mean, who wouldn't? Well, the lymph system's sole job and function is to see to it that such a life of well-being is a reality. *That's its job.* That's why it exists! It is, therefore, peculiar in the extreme, to put it mildly, that most of the people reading this cannot describe what their own body's lymph system is or what it does, even though it is the single most important factor in achieving and maintaining the highest level of health.

If you doubt what I'm saying about people not knowing what the lymph system is, I have a fun little experiment for you. After you finish reading the next few paragraphs, which will put you in a small minority of people who know exactly what the lymph system is, here's what you do: Start asking people, anyone you bump into, if they know what their body's lymph system is. What you will find is that most people don't have a clue. Some people say something like, "Sure I do, it's the . . . you know . . . the lymph system, right. It's in the body and has lymph nodes." Others will point to the side of their necks and say, "Yeah, there's one right here, right?" But most just scrunch up their brows as they contemplate the question and look at you as though you just asked them to name the nineteenth president. Now, if they say, "Yeah, it's the body's garbage collector in charge of keeping us alive and well," then you know they read this book or my last book, the entirety of which was on this very subject.[3]

> **A** human being is an ingenious assembly of portable plumbing.
>
> —CHRISTOPHER MORLEY

As a normal, natural, completely necessary course of events, the human body is *always* producing wastes, which are referred to as toxins. This isn't a bad thing; it's simply how the living body functions. If you think of the human body as a machine, you can compare it to a car. You put fuel in the car, and as you drive around, poisonous fumes are emitted from the exhaust pipe, and sludge accumulates in the oil. With the human machine, you exhale carbon dioxide with every breath, and waste accumulates in the lymph system. Even the most healthy people on Earth have some toxins in their bodies; they have to. These toxins are constantly being generated from two sources. The first is from spent cells. Every day, approximately 300 billion cells in your body die and are immediately replaced by new ones. The second source of toxins is from the residue of the approximately seventy tons of food that the body metabolizes in a lifetime. The spent cellular debris and food residue comprise these toxins, the wastes that must be removed from the body as quickly as possible so as not to cause harm. Enter the lymph system.

The lymph system's reason for being is to collect toxins, degrade them—break them down—and transport them to the bloodstream, which in turn carries them to the four channels of elimination: the bowels, bladder, lungs and skin. This all takes place with unsurpassed precision and proficiency. Problems only arise when the lymph system is burdened with more of these toxins than it can handle. In other words, when more wastes are generated than are eliminated, the toxins have to go somewhere, so they start to saturate the cells and all manner of health problems can result.

Do you know what happens to your car if you don't change the oil a few times a year? It becomes so silted up with sludge that the car will stop dead and not run. The lymph system also has to be kept clean and not be allowed to become overwhelmed, or it will become ineffective. And if that happens, look out, my friend, because you are in some deep trouble.

If removing toxins is the primary function of the lymph system and it's so good at it, how does it become overwhelmed in the first place? Like everything else concerning the activities of the living body, down to the last detail, it all has to do with energy. Don't forget, digestion is like the dominant lion at feeding time. Once he has had his fill, then and *only* then can the rest of the pride share what's left. Digestion *always* gets all the energy it needs to deal with food in the stomach, and whatever energy is remaining is divided amongst all the other activities that must be conducted that day. This, of course, includes the elimination of toxins. When these other activities are chronically shortchanged, uneliminated toxins are stored in the body until such time as there is sufficient energy to remove them. Over time, these uneliminated toxins start to wreak havoc in the body, resulting in all manner of health problems, anything from headaches to catastrophic disease.

The super-intelligent body, which is, at all times, striving for its own self-preservation and highest level of well-being, does not sit idly by and allow this to unfold without a fight. When the level of toxins in the body has reached the saturation point and health is about to be compromised, the survival mechanism kicks in and uses the most reliable and infallible tool in the arsenal to get your attention and make you aware of the impending danger. Guess what that tool is? It's something that you, me and virtually all people have experienced at one time or another in our lives. Give up? Pain!

Pain was not given thee merely to be miserable under; learn from it, turn it to account.

—THOMAS CARLYLE

When danger looms, the body doesn't call out your name and say, "Hey, you better watch out, my lymph system is backed up, and if it's not cleaned out pretty soon, you're going to pay." It would be swell if the body did that, but it doesn't. Instead, it gets your attention the most surefire way it can. Let me ask: Does pain get *your* attention?

Pain is the number-one health complaint in the United States.[4] Nine out of ten American adults say they experience some kind of pain on a regular basis. What a surprise. It is sad and unfortunate that most people don't realize what a truly important role pain plays in the grand scheme of things.

> Pain is part of the body's magic.
> It is the way the body transmits a sign to
> the brain that something is wrong.
>
> —Norman Cousins

Nothing in the universe happens in a haphazard way. Not a leaf falls from a tree without purpose. One of the most well-established facts of life is that we live in a cause-and-effect universe. Things don't just happen; they happen in an orderly fashion for a definite reason. So it is with pain. It may be difficult to view it as such, but pain is a friendly messenger, alerting us to a situation that will become progressively worse if not addressed. If we had been properly educated to understand this, and instructed on how to conduct ourselves in a manner that allowed the lymph system to catch up and clean out, the pain would go away because its purpose would have been served. But in the most classic response of attacking the messenger because we don't like the message, pain is viewed as the enemy, an attack on our well-being that demands a counter-attack. Instead of learning how to get out of the way and allow the lymph system to do what it does best, we go to war against pain, and what do you think is the weapon of choice? Drugs!

I'm not suggesting that if you have a splitting headache you shouldn't take something for it. I'm talking about the issue of pain and our response to it on a much larger scale. What if there was a way of living and eating that prevented the headache from occurring in the first place? That's what I'm talking about here. Drugs are a Band-Aid. They're for use *after* there's a problem. You don't put a Band-Aid on *before* you cut yourself, do you? Properly caring for your lymph system prevents problems before they happen. Drugs have one purpose and one purpose only. They are used to mask and deaden symptoms. There is not a single drug amongst the thousands and thousands in existence that fixes or heals *anything*. That's not what they're for. They are designed to trick you into thinking the cause of pain is gone when it's not. Removing the pain does not remove the problem. It only hides it from you. The tragedy is that over time, taking a drug for every ache and pain ultimately allows the problem to become catastrophic. Because the drugs only hide the pain, the original problem, which is a lymph system overburdened with toxins, becomes worse and worse. Plus, the drugs themselves are, one and all, toxic and add to the level of toxins in the body, further burdening the already-burdened lymph system. As the problem worsens, the body gallantly tries to exhibit that it needs help by doing the only thing it can do: sound the alarm with more intense pain. This, of course, is met with more and stronger drugs—just the way the pharmaceutical industry likes it. When the lymph system is clean and operating well, the cycle of pain and drugs is broken, and pain-free well-being becomes the dominant factor in your life—just the way God likes it.

> Most diseases are the result of
> medication which has been prescribed to
> relieve and take away a beneficent and
> warning symptom on the part of Nature.
>
> —ELBERT HUBBARD

It is not my intention to imply that people simply discontinue taking the medications their physicians have prescribed. Such discontinuation is a process that should be conducted in a slow, deliberate way and under the watchful eye of the prescribing physician. My intention is to encourage people to realize that, instead of always opting for drugs at the slightest provocation, they can avail themselves of other options, which are frequently less dangerous and more effective.

The classic example of this type of automatic medicating is giving antibiotics to children running a fever. Perfectly reasonable people become panic-stricken if their child develops a fever. It's off to the doctor for some antibiotics before the body burns itself up or causes brain damage. The suggestion that the intelligent human body would raise its own temperature until it caused brain damage is one of the most patently absurd contentions I have ever heard.

How something as inherently beneficial and corrective as a fever, which the body initiates to *protect* itself, has been so horribly misunderstood is a question for the ages. A fever mobilizes the body's defenses. When there is an emergency, such as an overaccumulation of toxins in the body, metabolism is accelerated by increasing the amount of heat available, thus enhancing the healing process. This process is controlled by the hypothalamus, which is sort of a human thermostat.

Metabolism consists of the absorption of nutrients and the elimination of wastes (toxins). The heat is necessary to accelerate the elimination of toxins, which have accumulated beyond the body's ability to tolerate them and beyond the body's ability to eliminate without some extraordinary modification (i.e., fever). Heat acts as a catalyst that causes the toxins to liquefy and pass into the bloodstream, where they are transported to the organs of elimination and thereby out of the body.

Temperature regulation is one of the most basic mechanisms of the human body. It is initiated by the body, controlled by the body, and intelligently and carefully utilized by the body as one of its primary defense techniques. Is it really so difficult to accept that such a fundamental mechanism as temperature regulation, something the body is involved in *every second of your life*, would be used as a tool to protect and preserve itself?

In my over thirty years of experience, I have never seen or even heard of a single person, young or old, who actually died from a fever, *unless* the fever patient was drugged with antibiotics. A fever is used to facilitate the elimination of toxins. In some instances the burden of a toxic drug, with its own inherent side effects adding to the already existing burden of excess toxins in the body, will injure or kill a fever patient. In other words, it's the drugs that killed and the fever that was blamed. Do you know the literal meaning of the word "antibiotic"? *Against life!*

Do not fear a fever. It is one of the most common and obvious means by which the intelligent body protects itself. A patient with a fever should take no drugs, eat very, very lightly (ideally, fresh fruit and juices exclusively), drink water, stay still, use cool (*not* cold) compresses on the forehead, chest and back of the neck, and allow the body to do what it is trying to do without interference. The fever will then accomplish its intended task and subside. This is an instance when drugs can only hurt.

You must be wondering, and rightly so, why, if a clean lymph system is so important to health, it is not more widely understood. The answer is money. There's no money in it. A clean lymph system prevents ill health *before* it happens. The entire health-care industry in the United States, which generates $1.3 trillion a year (that's $3.5 billion every day, weekends included),[5] entirely depends on treating people *after* they're sick. There are no products to sell that flush the lymph system and keep it clean. It's not as though after telling you how crucial it is to keep your lymph system in good condition that I tell you I have the only patented formula for rejuvenating the lymph system, and for $129.95 a month you, too, can be saved. The lymph system cleans itself; it doesn't have to be forced or coerced into doing so. Your heart doesn't have to be forced to beat. Your eyelids don't have to be forced to blink. Your stomach doesn't have to be forced to digest food.

The incredible living body automatically takes care of itself. If you cut your finger, you don't have to do anything for it to heal. The body immediately marshals its forces and knows exactly and precisely what to do and how to do it. In an extraordinary display of proficiency and sophistication unrivaled by any machine or manmade apparatus, the body unleashes its power. First it coagulates the blood. Then it forms a hard casing over the wound to protect it, while underneath, the cells and tissues are reattached. The hard casing falls off, and the wound is healed. What a masterpiece! So it is with your lymph system. The body will automatically, and without prompting, break down and flush toxins from your system if it is given the opportunity to do so, and providing the body with more living food creates that opportunity. So you don't have to do anything more than what you are already going to do to lose weight, and as a bonus, your health will improve as well. How's that for a good deal?

Two apparatuses that are immensely beneficial to increasing the efficiency of the lymph system are the rebounder and the inversion table.

The rebounder is a mini-trampoline, and gently bouncing on it for short periods of time subjects the body to a change in velocity and direction twice with each bounce. This in turn opens and closes the lymph valves, which stimulates the flow of lymph through the body. The rebounder is easy to use and yields tremendous benefits, making it one of the most effective and efficient forms of exercise around. I have been using a rebounder every day for more than twenty years. I presently use the REBOUNDAIR rebounder.

The inversion table is an amazingly lightweight apparatus upon which the body can lie flat with the ankles held in place, allowing movement from slightly past horizontal to fully upside down. Because gravity pulls everything down, the benefits of reversing that pull for short periods of time are too numerous to mention, but include dramatic improvement of both lymph and blood flow. I have been tilting myself upside down for one to two minutes a day for several years. When I began this regimen, I suffered from intense lower-back pain, the number-one health complaint of adults in America. The day I started using the Teeter brand inversion table, which healthfully stretches the spine, my lower-back pain disappeared as if by magic, never to return.

I strongly recommend your looking into both rebounders and inversion tables. For more information:

1-877-942-4492 or 1-877-215-1212 (toll-free)
www.fitforlifetime.com

2. **All for One—One for All.** Although the body does prioritize where it will allocate energy, it does not show favoritism. Everything is its favorite and is cared

for equally. So yes, the lymph system will perform at a higher efficiency as a result of raising the level of living food provided the body. But the same can be said for all the other systems of the body as well. This translates into greater well-being on every level. On the physical side there will be an across-the-board improvement, inside the body and out. All of the numerous activities that go on unseen inside your body will be performed with greater efficiency. The entire cardiovascular system will work better, supplying all the cells with oxygenated blood. In fact, the process of oxygenating the blood through the lungs will improve. All of the elimination organs and processes will improve. Indeed, *all* your organs will operate on a higher level. *Every* system will work better; I don't know how else to say it. Even the reproductive system's functioning will improve. I know of at least three couples over the years who were unable to have children for various reasons. Either her ovaries weren't producing or his sperm count was too low. They had gone to doctors for help with no success. After dramatically increasing the living-food content of their diets, they became pregnant and had children.

All your senses will become more acute. I have been told by people that their hearing and eyesight improved. Your hair and skin will become more radiant. I have known people who had purple bags under their eyes for years. After a matter of months, sometimes only weeks, they were completely cleared up. I could go on and on describing the improvements in all areas of people's lives that have been reported to me. Every component of the living body works in a marvelously cooperative way, every part helping every other part. When you reach out your hand and grasp something, it's a synergistic process. Your muscles and bones, ligaments and tendons, fingers and palm of the hand, all work together to seize an object and hold onto it. Everything works in harmony in one great effort of collaboration for the common good of the living body.

> A healthy body is a guest chamber
> for the soul; a sick body
> is a prison.
>
> —FRANCIS BACON

It doesn't end at the physical, either. The physical is only one part. You can think more clearly. Your emotions improve. A positiveness starts to permeate your life that affects every area of your being and existence. Physically, intellectually, emotionally and spiritually, your life is uplifted—all from the single act of increasing the amount of living food while decreasing the amount of cooked food in your diet.

I know very well that it all sounds a bit too good to be true. But that is only because of your conditioned thinking. Your living body is a miracle, and it is capable of doing miraculous things. I have watched far too many people have the results I'm referring to over the last thirty-plus years to doubt it for even a moment.

3. **Fuel for Life.** I have already spoken at length of the important role energy plays in our lives, and why not? Without it we can do nothing; our bodies can do nothing. When all energy is gone, our lives are over. In my nearly sixty times around the sun, I have never, ever heard people wish for less energy or complain that they had too much. Have you? We've all known people who either were dragging around all the time, complaining about not having enough energy to do the simplest things, or those who seemed to have so much energy that they're annoying. Some people, no matter what they're doing, seem to be pulling a piano behind them that is tethered to their waists. And there are those who are brimming over with enthusiasm, practically bouncing off the walls and suggesting all manner of activities—for fun! We pass them by and muse, "Whatever s/he's on, I want some." *Energy!* One of the most gratifying aspects of my work is seeing that certain sparkle in people's eyes when they enthusiastically express their delight with all of their newfound energy. I never tire of seeing it or hearing about it.

The world belongs to the energetic.
—ALEXIS DE TOCQUEVILLE

Starting in the 1990s, a term was used to describe a malady that has now become so prevalent that I doubt there is anyone who has not at least heard it mentioned. It's called chronic fatigue syndrome, and it is *not* fun, as anyone who suffers from it would certainly attest. Chronic fatigue syndrome is characterized primarily by overwhelming fatigue to the point where the individual can hardly function. Some of this syndrome's other symptoms are muscle weakness, sleep disturbances (either insomnia or increased sleep), headaches, joint pain, irritability, forgetfulness, confusion, difficulty thinking or poor concentration, depression and painful glands.

I am bringing up the subject because, in my opinion, chronic fatigue syndrome is about as classic an example as I can think of to illustrate the effect a prolonged diet predominated by cooked food can have in overwhelming the lymph system. It is *exactly* what I was referring to when I spoke of the overburdened lymph system storing toxins throughout the body until sufficient energy was made available to eliminate it. It is therefore not surprising in the least that painful glands are one of the symptoms. They're full of toxins! What further convinces me that I am right is the fact that anyone I know who has had chronic fatigue syndrome and was willing to start eating more living food and less cooked food made dramatic turnarounds.

The medical approach is almost laughable. It is believed that there is no known cause for chronic fatigue syndrome. The best guess is that it is the result of the biggest scapegoat in the history of the universe: a virus. Perhaps the herpes virus number six, or maybe an enterovirus, or maybe a retrovirus. Any time members of the medical community are completely dumbfounded and unable to shed even the slightest ray of light on a problem, they suggest that it must be a virus, which lets them off the hook. But even though there is supposedly no known cause, there *are* some experimental treatments, all having to do with, what else—drugs! Throw drugs at it. Why not? Maybe something will accidentally work. There's the antiviral drug, Zovirax. There are selected drugs that "adjust" the immune response, such as intravenous gammaglobulin Amphiagen and something called transfer factor. Then there are tricyclic antidepressants, histamine 2-blocking agents, such as Tagamet, and antianxiety agents, such as Xanax. The drugs never work because they don't address the cause, and, in fact, add their own toxins to the already struggling lymph system, compounding the problem.

Any time people regularly lack energy, either intermittently or chronically, as with chronic fatigue syndrome, you can bet that their digestive tract is working overtime, all the time. Truly, one of the most cherished benefits of eating as much living food as cooked food is the increased level of energy that those who do so are able to enjoy.

4. **Build It Strong.** As indicated earlier, we humans are here to eat—we're eating machines. The way the

living body is designed, we must eat in order to stay alive, and if we don't, we die. There is such a mind-boggling array of different foods to tempt us with such an endless variety of different flavors that we tend to lose sight of the single most important reason for eating. It is to supply the body with the building blocks of life: nutrients. These come from the vitamins, minerals, amino acids, fatty acids, antioxidants, and all other substances and compounds *known* and *unknown* that are carried into our bodies via the foods we eat. What a marvelously elegant and extraordinary process has been devised by the intelligence that constructed our bodies and gave us life! We actually remove organic matter from our environment, transfer it into our bodies and it *becomes* us. Wow! *Double-wow!* There is no way to begin to try to comprehend the indescribably complex actions involved in turning a foodstuff, which in no way, shape or form whatsoever resembles us, into blood, bone, skin, teeth, hair and organs. It's a process that we take totally for granted, but there isn't a scientist alive who could duplicate the process or explain how it's accomplished.

Knowledge is the small part of ignorance that we arrange and classify.

—AMBROSE BIERCE

There can never be a substitute that will furnish a human being with all of the nutritional elements required for superior health. We have come a long way in understanding the human body and the factors involved in nurturing it. Physiology books abound with thousands and thousands of salient facts that explain the numerous activities and processes of the amazing human machine. And if you were to combine absolutely everything that is known, it would be dwarfed by what is not known and is yet to be learned. We do not yet know all of the elements that are structural constituents of the body. There are what are called recommended daily allowances (RDAs) of nutrients, but they are nothing more than speculative guesses. We do not yet know for certain how much of any food element the body needs. Plenty of vitamins have been isolated and named, but we do not know that all vitamins have been discovered. In fact, there are very likely many more food factors that may be absolutely essential to life that are not yet known.

Here's what we *do* know: Our physiology has developed over hundreds of thousands of years, and our entire system is geared toward extracting the elements of life from plant foods. Certain high-quality supplements can *assist*, but they could never replace what we require from food. Only people with a vested interest will tell you differently.

Any time you hear of some spectacular new discovery of a substance in food that fights cancer or boosts the immune system or wards off Alzheimer's, where does it come from? A plant food! You never have, nor will you hear of some wonderful substance that in some way improves one's health that has been isolated in a pork chop.

What I want you to know is that by eating more living food you are fueling your body with the best of what it needs to function at its highest level, and you are supplying nutrients in their finest, most easily accessible and utilizable form. People sometimes ask me if it isn't true that the soil is so depleted that what we need isn't even in the food. More often than not you will hear that from someone trying to sell you something. It's *not* true. I'm not saying that the soil hasn't been compromised, but I'll tell you something interesting about this. Plants require certain prerequisites to sprout and grow. If they don't receive them from the sun, water and soil, they won't grow. The very constituents that the plants, once grown, contain are precisely what we need from the plant. Don't ever believe for a moment that there is anything superior to living food that will supply your body with what it needs to excel.

5. **Clean, Not Clogged.** I want to put something into perspective for you. You're familiar with 747 jumbo jets, are you not? They're so huge they even have a spiral staircase inside that goes to an upper level. Fully staffed and with every seat filled, the 747 carries about 500 people. If tragedy strikes and one of these behemoths goes down and everyone on board perishes, it is in the news for weeks, months, even years sometimes until the cause of the crash is determined. Investigations are ongoing, and the National Transportation

Safety Board (NTSB) relentlessly stays on it until all questions are answered. The true cost is, of course, the loss of life and the effect it has on the surviving loved ones of the 500 people. The pain of such a loss lasts long after the event. That is the effect of *one* of these planes going down.

Could you even begin to comprehend the effect of the equivalent number of people dying if *five* 747s went down every single day of the year without letup? It's too outrageous to even contemplate for a moment. That would be 2,500 people dying *every day*. As it happens, more people than that die every day from the biggest killer this country has ever known: cardiovascular disease. Cardiovascular disease is any disease having to do with the heart and some 90,000 miles of blood vessels. It includes heart attacks, strokes, atherosclerosis (accumulation of fatty deposits or fibrosis of the arterial walls), arteriosclerosis (thickening or hardening of the arterial walls) and any other disease of the heart and blood vessels. Cardiovascular disease takes so many lives that if you were to add up all deaths from all other causes of death by disease combined, they would not come close to equaling the number of deaths from cardiovascular disease alone. And here's something that should stop you in your tracks. Did you know that 98 percent of our children in the United States already have at least one symptom of heart disease?[6]

What happens is that the veins and arteries to and from the heart become clogged and blocked, and that's when the mischief starts. Do you know what the primary cause of this blockage is? Saturated fat and cholesterol. Cholesterol in particular has people in an uproar, as a result of the regular flow of items on the news reporting both on the danger cholesterol poses to health and the damage it continues to wreak. We've known this for some time. Back in 1990, the government's National Institutes of Health stated it clearly when it reported that, "The relation-ship between high blood cholesterol and heart dis-ease was undisputed and there were unequivocal benefits to reducing blood cholesterol levels."[7] The level of cholesterol in your blood is known as your "serum cholesterol." It is a measure of units of milli-grams of cholesterol per 100 milliliters of blood, or what is called milligram percent (mg%). A person with a cholesterol level of 260 mg% is five times more likely to die from a heart attack than one with a level of 200 mg%.[8] In the United States 200 mg% has become the benchmark, whereby if you're at or under 200 mg% you're okay, and if you're over 200 mg% you're at risk. The average person in the United States is definitely over 200 mg%.

It is for this reason that products abound in the marketplace that either declare there is no cholesterol contained in them or that they will in some way lower cholesterol. It goes without saying that there are drugs galore that promise to lower cholesterol, but as is the case with all drugs, they have negative side effects, including the ultimate negative side effect of death.

I remember a simpler time. Back in the late 1960s and early 1970s, if a man wanted to strike up a conversation with a woman, all he had to say was, "Hi, my name's Bob. I'm an Aquarius, what's *your* sign?" That was all it took. The conversation would flow from that opening as though the two were old friends. It's just a wee bit different today, though. Today it is more like, "Hi, my name's Bob. I'm HIV negative and my cholesterol is under 200." Of course, this means that Bob can have sex and won't drop dead of a heart attack.

I find it strange that after all this time some people are still confused about where cholesterol comes from, especially since it comes from only one place in the universe and absolutely nowhere else. Cholesterol is produced in the livers of animals. In fact, we human beings produce about 1,000 mg of cholesterol *every day*. That is because cholesterol is a necessity of life. Practically every function of the body, from blinking the eyes to swallowing, from walking to internal functions, requires cholesterol. However, it's not the cholesterol the body produces for its own use and well-being that presents any problem; it's the cholesterol from other animals we eat that is the culprit. There's no such thing as cholesterol coming from nuts or avocados or any other plant food—or, for that matter, any place other than the liver of animals. Period. So the less animal products people eat, the less harmful cholesterol they take in. The more animal products people eat, the more cholesterol they ingest. It is unlikely in the extreme that you will ever hear of a vegetarian having elevated cholesterol levels, because they don't eat animal products.

Some advertisers prey on the confusion by advertising their products with a big "NO CHOLESTEROL" when there's no way cholesterol could be in the product in the first place unless it was intentionally added. The other day I saw an ad on TV that was advertising cans of mixed nuts, and it made a point of saying, "And there's no cholesterol." They might as well have added, "And there's no cigarette butts," because there's no way it could contain them either, unless they were added. Or how about no rat poison or razor blades? The only way the can of nuts could contain cholesterol is if they mixed in some chopped-up pieces of liver.

What I can tell you is that by increasing the amount of living food in your diet while decreasing the amount of cooked food, including animal products even to a small degree, the only possible result, as concerns harmful cholesterol, is that you will have less of it in your blood.

6. **The Fiber Con.** I have a riddle for you. What is it that *everyone* wants? Looks forward to? And feels wonderful with and lousy without, yet is rarely, if ever, spoken about? Let me give you just a moment to think about it. Okay, did you figure it out? Bowel movements! Am I right? My friend Mr. Bremmer, whom I spoke of earlier, once said to me (remember, he was in his eighties), "Let me tell you something, Sonny, the older you get the more you'll come to realize that there's nothing in life quite like waking

up in the morning and having a good bowel movement." His language was a bit more colorful to be sure, but I think you get the point.

What a sad and telling commentary it is that so many constipated people have been reduced to spending hundreds of millions of dollars every year on laxatives because they are unable to have something as natural and normal as regular bowel movements. The elimination of wastes from the body *should* be easier than throwing a rock into a lake. After all, for its very survival, the living body *must, wants to* and *will* eliminate wastes—provided that it is not clogged up as a result of the wrong type of diet, namely one that is sorely lacking in or devoid of dietary fiber. Fiber is the key.

Fiber is found *only* in plants. It is the tough, chewy part of fruit, vegetables, nuts, seeds and grains. It is what gives structure to plants. Fiber cannot be digested by humans because it resists digestive enzymes. The best way to obtain the finest fiber is by eating uncooked, living foods in their natural state. The use of refined, cooked foods and the consequent lack of dietary fiber lead to pathological problems, especially in the digestive tract. Fiber is absolutely necessary for sufficient digestion. Fiber also absorbs fat and harmful substances and thus prevents their absorption into the blood. The properties of fiber also help remove harmful chemicals from the body and reduce levels of cholesterol. And, of course, adequate dietary fiber is what produces more frequent and more thorough bowel movements, thus removing wastes before they can cause disease.

> The most costly of all follies is to believe passionately in the palpably not true.
>
> —H. L. Mencken

The cashectomist is a Johnny-on-the-spot who will con you into buying all manner of hatched-up, chemical-laden concoctions with slick ads that tell you how easy and convenient it now is to get your fiber. Of course, you're not told that it's far easier on your wallet, and on your health, to *eat some fruit or a salad!* In one study referred to in the journal *Lancet*, researchers found that "precancerous growths, or polyps, were slightly more likely to recur in those taking a certain fiber supplement."[9] At the end of the article, it was recommended that "a low-fat, high-fiber diet rich in fruits and vegetables" be eaten for fiber. What do you know? I am somewhat encouraged to some truth in advertising in one product that comes right out and calls itself FiberCon.

> Live all you can; it's a mistake not to. It doesn't so much matter what you do in particular, so long as you have your life. If you haven't had that, what *have* you had?
>
> —Henry James

7. **The Ultimate Gift.** Truly, there is no greater gift than life. And a *long* life is the most cherished. When I speak of a long life I am most certainly not talking about one riddled with pain and ill health, or length of life at any cost, even if that means being confined to a bed with tubes from the body connected to machines in order to prolong life. I'm talking about a long, productive life of vibrancy.

If you were to ask people at random to list what they thought were the foremost keys to a long life, I wonder how many of them would mention successfully streamlining the digestive process. It's not what first pops into mind, is it? Most people have literally no idea that there is not a casual, but a *direct,* link between long life and the efficiency of their digestive tracts.

We know we must eat to stay alive; that's a given. And the entire process of eating seventy tons of food in a lifetime, breaking it down and digesting it, extracting what is needed from it and eliminating the waste requires more life energy than all other uses of energy combined. Unquestionably, other factors are involved in achieving long life; I'm not suggesting there aren't. What I *am* suggesting is that a well-working digestive system is right up there, close to or at the top of the list.

I'm going to tell you about a gentleman I have written and talked about many times in the past. He is someone whose work has been instrumental in bringing to light an awareness of the vital link between facilitating the digestive process and long life. His name is Roy Walford, M.D. Dr. Walford is considered one of the world's most eminent gerontologists. He was head of a large research laboratory at UCLA, a member of both the White House Conference on Aging and of the National Academy of Science's Committee on Aging, as well as chairman of the National Institute on Aging Task Force, and has written several books on the subject. In other words, he knows what he's talking about when it comes to the subject of long life and what supports it.

Dr. Walford's notoriety stems, to a great extent, from his work with mice. You see, the average life span of mice is about two years. But the mice in Dr. Walford's experiments all lived twice that long. He's figured out how to *double* their life span. Plus, the longer-living mice have fewer degenerative diseases than the mice living half as long. Quite a feat, wouldn't you agree? How did he do it? It wasn't with some magical formula, not with some rare, exotic substance or obscure and mysterious treatment. He doubled their life spans by completely resting their digestive tracts for two days a week. That's the long and short of it. By fasting his mice two days a week and giving them only water so as to require no energy being spent on digestion, he doubled the length of their lives. Dr. Walford, now in his late seventies, is quick to point out that he fasts two days a week.

Perhaps you can see why I place such a strong emphasis on doing whatever possible to ease the work of your digestive tract. The entirety of the approach to losing weight that I am putting forth in this book is based on streamlining the digestive process. Many health benefits in addition to losing weight accrue from eating more living food, from less pain and disease to more energy and general well-being. But in the long run, looking at the big picture, surely its greatest appeal has to be its implications for longevity.

Someday I would like to stand on the moon, look down through a quarter of a million miles of space and say, "There certainly is a beautiful Earth out tonight."

—Lt. Col. William H. Rankin

---

8. **Eartheart.** This last benefit to your life that I'm going to share with you is on a much grander scale and has a much more far-reaching effect on the world around you than do the ones already listed. When most people sit down to a meal, they have a general idea that the food they're about to eat is going to have an effect on their life on Earth. There are very few people, however, who have even an inkling of an idea how their food choices are going to affect the life *of* Earth.

A few pages ago I laid out the devastating effect that eating animal products can have on the heart because of the cholesterol that all animal products contain. What would you think if I were to tell you that our love affair with animal products has a similar devastating effect on the environment of our planet? The same thing that is devastating so many hearts is also contributing to the destruction of the Earth. And as a *not* coincidental exclamation point to that statement, consider that if you take the *h* from the front of the word "heart," and place it at the end of the word, you have the word "Earth." Earth and heart are the same word depending upon where the *h* is placed.

I think it's reasonable to say that most people are aware that our environment has been somewhat compromised and if there was some simple act they could perform that would improve it, they would. After all, our children and our children's children will have to live in the future with whatever decisions our generation makes today.

> Now there is one outstandingly important fact regarding Spaceship Earth, and that is that no instruction book came with it.
>
> —BUCKMINSTER FULLER

I think it's also safe to say that considering the magnitude of the challenge to "fix" the environment, each of us as individuals can't help but feel intimidated by the scope of the problem and powerless to make any real change. After all, we're talking about water pollution, air pollution, soil erosion, deforestation, the burning of fossil fuels and the depletion of our natural resources. Even for those who *want* to do their part, what can they do? Even if they had the time, between earning a living and taking care of their families, what can one person actually accomplish? I'm going to show you how, by taking the steps recommended in this book to lose weight and improve your health, you are simultaneously going to be making a significant contribution to healing the Earth. You don't have to write your congressperson; you don't have to march in the streets carrying placards; you don't have to hand out flyers. It's all done at the dinner table with your knife and fork.

If you are anything like most of the people to whom I've brought up this subject, you are wondering something like, *What in the world does my cholesterol level have to do with the environment?* Just this: Have you ever stopped to think how many animals are eaten in the United States each year? Brace yourself: 6 billion.[10] That's 16 million every day, including cows, chickens, hogs, and various and sundry others such as sheep, rabbits, deer, etc. That's right: 16 million a day. Plus we also eat 165 million eggs, 11 million pounds of fish and 345 million pounds of dairy every single day.[11]

Can you even begin to imagine the amount of food it takes to feed 6 billion animals? Try to contemplate for a moment the resources that have to be used to plant, grow and harvest the food to feed 6 billion animals. Then they have to be fed. Then they are transported, slaughtered, packaged, stored and distributed. As you will see, the chain of events that unfolds from the time an animal is born until it winds up on your dinner plate appears to be designed specifically for the purpose of squandering our natural resources.

First, let's look at the land. When our founding fathers established the good ol' U.S. of A., 225 years ago, crop land had on average about twenty-one inches of top soil in which to grow our food. Today there are six inches remaining.[12] We lose another inch every twenty years, but it takes Mother Nature about 350 years to build just one inch of topsoil.[13] "So what?" you may say. "We gotta eat!" True enough. But a mere 5 percent of all land to grow food is used to grow the food eaten by humans. The other 95 percent of all the land is used to grow food to feed animals.[14] It requires over 500 times as much land to produce a pound of beef than a pound of produce.[15] The most plentiful crop grown in America is corn. Of the total amount of corn eaten, almost 90 percent is consumed by livestock.[16] Most of the oats, rye, barely, sorghum and soybeans grown in the United States are fed to livestock as well. Also, when we first came to America, most of it was trees. The vast majority of the forest land that has been cleared was used for grazing livestock or for growing livestock feed.[17]

> How inappropriate to call this planet
> Earth, when it is clearly Ocean.
> —Arthur C. Clarke

Try to comprehend the amount of water necessary to grow all this food. A nearly incomprehensible amount of water is required. Trillions and trillions of gallons. There's only a fixed amount of water available to us. A certain amount of it will be used, and a certain amount of what's left will be polluted. More than half the water consumed in the United States is used in animal agriculture, most of which goes to irrigate land growing feed for livestock.[18] This is more water than all other industries combined. Mind you, the animal-products industry doesn't just use more than any other industry; it uses more than all other industries *combined*. Enough water goes into the production of one steer to float a U.S. naval destroyer.[19] The growing of one pound of wheat requires only 25 gallons of water, while the production of one pound of meat requires 2,500 gallons.[20] And what about the water that's left? The animal-products industry is responsible for the pollution of more water than all other industries combined.[21] Once again, not just more than any other industry, but more than all other industries *combined*. Not only is this from the millions of tons of pesticides that find their way into the water supply, but also *every second* 250,000 pounds of excrement is produced by livestock in our country for which there is no sewage system.[22] So most of it finds its way into our water. Astonishingly, the U.S. Department of Agriculture used to have a policy of encouraging beef producers to situate feedlots on hillsides near streams to facilitate the easy channeling of waste into the water.[23] Yuck.

Then there's the energy connection. Where is all this energy being used? When you drive down the highway behind a huge truck belching out thick plumes of black smoke, it's easy to make the connection between moving vehicles, energy usage and carbon-dioxide pollutants in the air. But ask people to make a connection between energy usage and sitting down to a breakfast of bacon and eggs, a hamburger for lunch or a steak dinner and they can't see the association. There are fleets of farm equipment, tractors and farm trucks in constant use performing the day-to-day activities of running thousands of farms. The vehicles used to plow and till the soil, spread fertilizer, spray pesticides, haul away the prodigious amount of wastes and perform other farm chores are some of the least fuel-efficient vehicles and equipment in existence. They get perhaps a mile or two a gallon. Plus there's the carbon dioxide. Right at this moment, trucks and trains are criss-crossing this country with livestock animals. Cattle, for example, are transported from the farms to the feeding lots to the auction houses to the finishing lots to the slaughterhouses and then to the distribution centers for sale to the public. Once again, trucks and trains are some of the least fuel-efficient means of travel.

The main ingredient for the fertilizers used on crops is nitrogen, and natural gas is required for its production. Twenty billion pounds of nitrogen is used a year.[24] The natural gas used to make fertilizer is enough to fuel all the gas-burning stoves, ovens and other gas-burning appliances in the country. Plus there's the energy necessary for all the refrigeration required to keep 6 billion animal parts from decomposing from the time the animal is slaughtered until you buy it at the supermarket. All told, the energy requirements of the animal-products industry represents a titanic, unrelenting drain on our country's energy resources while adding its share of pollutants into the air.

The world is disgracefully managed.
One hardly knows to whom
to complain.

—RONALD FIRBANK

I could go on and on, believe me, but the point has been made. I suspect that the next time you hear someone having difficulty connecting the eating of a hamburger to the crises with the environment, you'll hardly know where to begin.

Let me now describe the effects of a mere 10 percent reduction of animal-product usage in the United States alone. As an example, if there are twenty-one meals eaten a week (three meals times seven days) and at least some animal products are eaten at all of them, a 10 percent reduction would be achieved by simply having no animal products at two of those twenty-one meals. That seemingly insignificant effort, if carried out by the population of the United States, would have a mind-boggling effect. Hold on to your hats. Over 1.5 *trillion* gallons of pure water will be saved a year.[25] That is equivalent to over 3 million gallons of precious water being saved every minute of every hour of every day of the year. Nearly one-half trillion pounds of animal excrement a year will not be dumped into our waterways.[26] The reduced need for fuel will lower fossil-fuel demand by the equivalent of 2.3 billion gallons a year.[27] That's a savings of over 6 million gallons a day. Seven hundred million tons of topsoil will be saved a year.[28] Six hundred million animals a year would be saved from the slaughterhouse.[29] And as a final plus for which there can be no price attached, consider this: Every year the world over, 20 million people die of starvation and starvation-related diseases. That's someone dying of starvation every one and a half seconds without stop. A 10 percent reduction of animal-product usage in the United States would free up 12 million tons of grain, enough to feed every one of those 20 million people.[30] There are those who would say that even if the food were freed up, there are political, transportation and financial considerations that may prevent the food from reaching the people. True. But at least they would have a *chance* of receiving it. There is *no* chance if it's all fed to livestock.

The least movement is of importance
to all nature. The entire ocean
is affected by a pebble.

—BLAISE PASCAL

So many people feel that their single voice is too small to be heard, that their efforts would be too little to make any real difference. To paraphrase Edmund Burke, "No greater mistake could be made in life than doing nothing because you could only do a little." When a lot of people do a little, it's a *lot*. When a lot of people do nothing, it's *nothing*. If you decide to eat according to the principle of at least 50 percent of your diet being comprised of living food, you will, of necessity, be lowering your intake of animal products at least 10 percent. You will not only be helping yourself live a longer, healthier life, but you will also, admirably, be helping your country and the world, making you in the truest sense a caring and concerned citizen of the Earth.

CHAPTER EIGHT

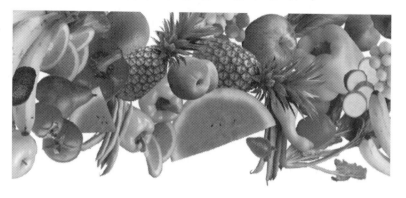

THE LONG
AND WINDING ROAD

It is difficult to say what is impossible,
for the dream of yesterday is the
hope of today and reality
of tomorrow.

—Robert Goddard

I feel compelled to share something with you. Testimonials always seem to make a difference to people who are interested in trying something new. To hear of someone's success lends credence to whatever is being considered, plus it gives you confidence knowing it's been tried and proved by someone else. I won't have to check the facts about this particular testimonial because it's my own.

I have earlier spoken of my own health problems that led me to dedicate myself to the study of health and how to achieve it: the stomachaches, the headaches, being overweight and watching my dad die of complications of stomach cancer. Although I definitely hated being fat, the stomachaches were, in particular, the most painful and disruptive of my personal ills. I could never fully describe the torture of being in constant pain, forced to double over to try to lessen the effect. This was from the time I was three years old until twenty-five years old. All the doctors would say was I had a "delicate stomach." Many times as a youngster I wouldn't tell my folks how bad it was, or they might make me swallow some of that abysmal Pepto-Bismol, which to me was nearly as bad as the pain itself. I didn't participate in sports; I rarely went on dates; I didn't have the energy for anything. This was topped off by watching my dad die of cancer of the stomach after complaining of the very same stomach pains that I had.

By the time I met the person who introduced me to

Natural Hygiene, the field of study *based* on eating living food, I was ready to try anything. I would have dueled the devil with burning pitchforks if I thought it would help. This person told me in such a matter-of-fact way that all my ills and overweight condition were because I ate a diet of nearly *all* dead food that I couldn't help but want to try it and see for myself. My recovery and return to health were so swift and so complete that I was consumed with the desire to learn all I possibly could about the subject of Natural Hygiene, and then make it my business to "spread the word." As part of my reward for doing so, I have not had a stomachache for over thirty years.

On numerous occasions in the past when I have been reading a book or listening to a tape or talking to someone I admire on the subject of our spiritual nature, one particular point of view has been raised that never fails to intrigue me. It revolves around seeing something good in the worst of situations. No matter how bad something is, it always has a spark of good if you are willing to see it. Or it can be stated a different way: Everything happens for the best, even though you can't always see it while in the midst of pain and suffering. I've always had a great respect for those who could maintain such a high-minded and lofty way of viewing the world. I have, over the years, endeavored to imbibe such an elevated way of thinking, and I can see that some of my own past difficulties were indeed necessary in order to bring me to my next level of evolution.

As much as I suffered with and cursed those stomach-aches, they led me to Natural Hygiene, without which I don't know what my health would be like today or if I would even be alive. Plus, literally millions of people have also benefited from what they learned about Natural Hygiene in the books I have written—books that I could not possibly have written had my own ill health not been such a motivating influence in my life. But it wasn't until much, much later—some twenty years after discovering Natural Hygiene—that the full impact of the good that sprang forth from the not-so-good became clear to me.

In 1966, when I was twenty-one years old, I was in the U.S. Air Force, having enlisted three years earlier right out of high school in order to fulfill my obligation to the country while I was young. The war was raging in Vietnam, and as fate would have it, I was sent there for a one-year tour of duty. I won't lie to you: I was scared to death of going there and actually being put into the position of having to shoot and kill another human being. I had never even held a weapon in my hand before entering the service. But, thank the Lord in heaven, I never had to fire my weapon, and my stay there was relatively uneventful, especially compared to friends of mine who were put to the ultimate test. Some survived; some didn't.

In 1967, I was sent home and honorably discharged. I was overwhelmingly elated that I made it home safe and unscathed. The '60s were in full bloom, and I dove right in and went on a three-and-a-half-year party, which for me meant eating anything I could fit in my mouth. Of course the result was that I ballooned up to over 200 pounds and severely compromised my health.

It was 1970 when I discovered the information I have been relating to you in this book. I lost my weight, got my health in order, studied Natural Hygiene like a man possessed, and *Fit for Life* was published in 1985. It became an instant sensation, and by the beginning of 1986 I was on top of the world. *Fit for Life* was number one on all the best-seller lists, and I was in heaven. But I was in for the shock of my life. It turns out that I did *not* make it home unscathed from Vietnam. What I didn't know was that I had been exposed, over and over again, to Agent Orange while I was there.

Dioxin is a byproduct of Agent Orange and is the most toxic man-made chemical ever concocted. It's a thousand times stronger than the strongest weed killer. It was used in an attempt to defoliate the country of all its jungles so there would be nowhere to hide. Between 1962 and 1971, 11 million gallons were sprayed. It didn't work. When it was being sprayed, it was thought to be harmless to human beings, but that was before it was discovered that the poison sits in the body for twenty years before there is any indication of its harmfulness. There's a long list of devastating ailments caused by Agent Orange poisoning, one of which is called peripheral neuropathy, and it is the one that presently has me in its grip.

Peripheral neuropathy causes the wasting away of muscles. It usually starts in the arms and legs, then spreads to the body. Five years after deterioration starts (which, remember, is twenty years after exposure), those who are not dead are immobilized in a wheelchair, unable to move. It has now been seventeen years since I started losing muscle in my arms and legs, making me one of the longest-known survivors to still be walking around on his own without assistance. I do have obvious, lingering damage in that I limp noticeably, and have to struggle with both arms and both hands to accomplish the simplest tasks that even a small child could easily accomplish with one hand. But, I'm alive! And notwithstanding the damage to my limbs, I am in excellent health.

I was exposed to Agent Orange in 1966, and my muscles started to atrophy in 1986, twenty years to the day. The reason I am alive and perhaps the longest-known survivor is because I was led to the importance of eating living food in 1970, which was only four years after exposure. That enabled my lymph system to have a fighting chance against Agent Orange. The way I look at it is, if I wasn't overweight and suffering from violent stomachaches, I probably would not have discovered the importance of eating living food, and I wouldn't even be here right now. So you see, good can come out of even dire circumstances, depending on your point of view.

There's no such thing as chance;
and what to us seems merest accident
springs from the deepest
source of destiny.

—FRIEDRICH VON SCHILLER

I happen to have a positive outlook on life. I refuse to allow negative thinking to rule me. As far as I'm concerned, we are all children of a loving God who wants us to be happy and fulfilled. No matter what tribulations befall us, all are the result of God working in our lives for our greater good. I can't say exactly why, after studying how to be healthy for most of my life, I am saddled with peripheral neuropathy, but it's not my job to try to second-guess God. Perhaps it's so I will be more understanding of those facing tremendous challenges. Perhaps it's to be the living example of what I'm setting forth in this book.

Maybe you can see the reason for my over-the-top enthusiasm for eating living food. And the purpose of my sharing this story with you should be glaringly obvious. It is my contention that uneliminated toxins are a major contributing factor to being overweight—and to being sick. Living food allows the body to keep the level of toxins to a minimum so as not to cause these problems. If I can come out victorious over the most deadly toxin ever made, do you see that you, with only the naturally occurring, run-of-the-mill toxins to deal with, can also be successful? You don't have to deal with dioxin; you only have to remove the residue of spent cells and the food you eat. Your body is supremely capable of doing this if it is properly fueled.

CHAPTER NINE

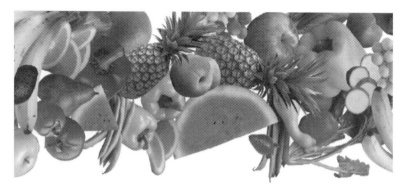

THE STUFF OF LIFE

Happiness is not a reward—
it is a consequence. Suffering is not a
punishment—it is a result.

—Robert Ingersall

Having made it to this point in the book, surely there can be no doubt in your mind that the goal of shedding excess weight and keeping it off long-term becomes a reality when weight loss becomes a way of living and eating that honors life, the living planet, your living body and living food. Throughout the book I have discussed the crucial role of enzymes, most notably in the food that must be eaten in order to stay alive. Once enzymes are destroyed by the heat of cooking, food is rendered lifeless, which affects your goal of losing weight and your well-being in two notable ways. First, the nutrients required to carry out all the processes and functions of the body are destroyed. Second, and perhaps even more important, is the tremendous extra burden placed on the digestive process, which as you know, has a direct impact on the amount of energy available to fuel all the body's many activities.

There are three categories of enzymes that have a direct influence in your life. First are food enzymes, which exist in all foods and assist in the breaking down of that food once inside the body. Second are digestive enzymes, which the body *must* produce for itself when food enzymes have been destroyed by cooking. Third are metabolic enzymes, which I have not mentioned until now, but which are without doubt the single most important factor you will ever learn about concerning the length and quality of your life—more important than anything you have learned thus far in this book.

Metabolic enzymes are the body's labor force. What do I mean by that? Literally every activity of your body depends upon, and is conducted by, metabolic enzymes. It is because of these wondrous little chemical protein powerhouses that you are able to swallow, breathe, blink your eyes, walk, talk, circulate blood—everything! You could not digest food, cleanse toxins from your lymph system or roll over in bed at night without the actions of metabolic enzymes. No one disputes the need to obtain the full complement of nutrients required for life. Without the activities of metabolic enzymes, those nutrients would never find their way to the cells for use. The reason you are alive is because of metabolic enzymes.

What you should know is that there is not a limitless supply of metabolic enzymes available to you. The human body has the capacity to manufacture only a certain number of them. A finite amount can be produced, and there is nothing under the sun that can force the body to make more once its capacity to do so has been exhausted. The inescapable truth of the matter is, you, I, everyone *will* run out of them at some point. And when there are no more metabolic enzymes, there is no more life. All of us will, at some point, come to the end of our lives, which in most cases means we have come to the end of our supply of metabolic enzymes. That may be at age 80 or 90 or 120, but the day will come. Whether a person dies from natural causes or from some disease, no matter what it states as the cause of death on the death certificate, the real and true cause is that there were no more metabolic enzymes available to carry out the functions of life, so life ended.

So the equation is a simple one: The more metabolic enzymes you require and use up, the shorter your life will be. The fewer metabolic enzymes you require and use up, the longer your life will be. And of that, there is simply no doubt. Therefore, it hardly seems necessary to say that *any-thing* that can be done to conserve what metabolic enzymes are available has to be the wisest, most intelligent course of action *ever*.

We know there is no way to force the body to make *more* metabolic enzymes, but what if there was a way to cause the body to use fewer of them? Guess what? *There is!* Haven't I mentioned innumerable times all throughout this book the vital and decisive role digestion plays in our lives and on our health? Nothing can help you achieve your health goals more quickly, whether it is to lose weight or to achieve a higher degree of overall health, than to stream-line the digestive process and free up energy for the purpose of cleansing the body. What do you think the effect is on the body when foods are eaten that have had all their enzymes destroyed by cooking? Since food in the stomach is a priority that cannot be ignored, the body must produce, on the spot, the enzymes necessary to digest it. There is no alternative to this; food cannot simply sit around in the stomach undigested. And guess where these enzymes that are produced to digest the food come from? From the only place they *can* come from—they are taken directly from the precious storehouse of metabolic enzymes, thus decreasing the amount available for all the activities that extend life.

We all are born with the ability to make a set amount of enzymes in our lifetimes, either digestive enzymes or metabolic enzymes. So every time any amount of cooked food is eaten, in the most literal sense possible, length of life is shortened because the more digestive enzymes the body is called upon to manufacture, the less metabolic enzymes will be able to be produced.

This fact used to prey on my mind every time I ate cooked food. So much so that for over a year straight, I ate exclusively living food. I felt incredible during that time, and it surely helped my body deal with the Agent Orange poisoning, for which I am eternally grateful. But even though I knew intellectually that it was the healthiest way to eat, there was no way I wanted to live out my life never eating cooked food again. I simply love to eat too much to entertain that idea. The next best thing was to set my sights on eating twice as much living food as cooked food, or two-thirds living and one-third cooked, which I have maintained to this day. That way I can enjoy all the cooked foods I like so as not to feel deprived and still know that the preponderance of what I am eating is nurturing and fueling my body. Still, I never stopped wishing for a way to eat cooked food that would not deplete my invaluable metabolic enzyme storehouse.

Then in 1995, with what was nothing short of an answer to prayer, my wish was granted. It was as though I found out there really *was* a Santa Claus, and he was bringing me the one thing I wanted more than anything else. Thanks to technological advances, a level of sophistication in understanding the structure and action of enzymes was reached, and Live Plant Enzymes were being produced and brought to market. Live Plant Enzymes are tiny capsules of plant-based digestive enzymes that are taken just prior to eating any cooked food, and they perform the function that the enzymes were supposed to perform before they were cooked away. I was in heaven at the prospect. I immediately started to research and study everything I could get my hands on about Live Plant Enzymes. It was all true. I have been taking Live Plant Enzymes with my cooked meals ever since, and they have been a great blessing in my life.

I've never been very keen on taking supplements; I'm just not a big pill-taker. During the height of *Fit for Life*'s popularity, I could have put my name on and recommended literally hundreds of products, but I chose to focus instead on the body's ability to excel when provided with the proper fuel for living, which is living food. But I'm not so stubborn and inflexible that I can't recognize something of tremendous worth when I see it. Every so often something comes along, a product of such inestimable worth and value, that the good it can provide cannot be denied. Such is the case with Live Plant Enzymes.

Here, in a nutshell, is what I can tell you about Live Plant Enzymes. They are pharmaceutical-grade and formulated under the most pristine conditions possible, in a laboratory setting without heat or chemicals. They are derived totally from a plant source, are 100 percent natural and organic, and have zero negative side effects. They come in tiny little capsules that are themselves plant-based so there is no chance of animal-borne contamination (E. coli, salmonella, mad cow disease, etc.).

By taking Live Plant Enzymes immediately before eating any cooked food, two immensely beneficial outcomes are realized, both of which have far-reaching positive effects as a result. First and foremost, it prevents the unnecessary squandering of metabolic enzymes, which in turn prolongs life. Since digestion always takes precedence over nearly everything else, many body functions requiring metabolic enzymes are often shortchanged during these times. The result is a general weakening of the body's ability to mend itself. Over time, this starts to take its toll, so it's harder to cleanse the body, remove wastes and lose weight.

To eat is human; to digest, divine.

—C. T. COPELAND

Second, Live Plant Enzymes increase the speed and thoroughness of digestion. As you must have gleaned from what you have read thus far, the very *last* thing you want to do is slow down digestion. On the contrary, anything that can streamline and make the digestive process more effective should always be the goal. Whether you are taking Live Plant Enzymes or not, the digestive tract and organs will always produce a certain number of digestive enzymes. But the body depends very much on the enzymes that are inherent in food to do its share of the work. When enzymes are missing in food because of cooking, the full burden of digestion falls on one's own enzyme-producing capacity, which not only overworks the digestive system but also causes a lag time for the food in the stomach while the body manufactures the enzymes it needs. Once again, over time we use up so much of our enzyme potential in making the digestive enzymes necessary to digest food that we begin to run short, and the ability to keep up with the digestive enzyme requirements begins to suffer. Poorly digested protein putrefies, fats turn rancid and starches ferment. This inevitably leads to malabsorption and poor nutrition and ultimately contributes to the long list of digestive disorders suffered by so many millions of people. Live Plant Enzymes are instrumental in preventing these problems *before* they occur. There is simply no price that can be put on the life-enhancing benefits of Live Plant Enzymes. In my opinion, the ability to make them is one of, if not the most significant and beneficial advances of the twentieth century in terms of the effect they can have on the length and quality of life.

An entire multibillion-dollar industry has been set up to treat the effects of disorders of the digestive system. Gas, bloating, indigestion, stomachaches, heartburn, acid reflux—*all* are the result of dietary indiscretions and an ineffective digestive tract. Drugs to quell the pain and discomfort of digestive disorders are the pharmaceutical industry's biggest moneymakers. It's the proverbial goose that lays the golden egg. Ever hear of the little purple pill, Prilosec? Unless you *never* watch TV, you have certainly seen the ads for it. It seems like you can't watch TV anymore without being pummeled with ads for drugs that are slick, beautiful to look at and designed to herald the industry's latest gumdrop. And after regaling you with how they can end your particular problem, they all end with the possible side effects that sometimes sound like you'd be better off being worked over with a tire iron and thrown down a flight of concrete stairs. By law, all such ads must give the most common side effects. You can bet your house they wouldn't do so if it were not mandated. This is the tricky part, as they don't want to scare anyone off. So they don't show a picture of a bloody ulcer, or someone holding their aching head, or doubled over with abdominal pain, or running to the nearest bathroom. No, the beautiful images remain before your eyes while someone casually, almost as an afterthought, gleefully mentions the bad news. Of course it's worded to minimize what can happen to you while giving you the overall impression that it's basically something as safe as a stroll on the beach.

The little purple pill is for heartburn. The ads all give a toll-free number for more information, so I called and had their promotional package sent. A beautiful full-color brochure showed up to tell me that I probably wasn't actually suffering from heartburn, but rather a brand-spanking-new disease called gastroesophageal reflux disease (GERD), for which the makers, AstraZeneca, just happen to have the remedy. I remember hearing at the end of the TV ad that the most common side effects were headache, abdominal pain and diarrhea. At the time I wondered who in the world would want to trade in some heartburn for a headache, stomachache *and* diarrhea? And on top of that, pay money for the privilege! I decided to see what the full list of possible side effects were.

In the package sent to me along with the beautiful

brochure was a four-page insert. This one, however, wasn't pretty at all. In fact, it was straight black-on-white, and all four pages were covered, top to bottom, with the tiniest print I've ever seen. My regular reading glasses were insufficient to read it so I had to use a magnifying glass. On the back page was a section called "adverse reactions," which is a list of *all* the possible side effects, not only the most common ones, which is all that *legally* has to be mentioned in the ads. *Oh, my God!* It was while reading the *full* list of possible side effects that I knew I must tell this tale. Now you'll see why AstraZeneca chose to tell you of them *only* in print so small you need a magnifying glass to read it.

Hold on to your hat because here's the full list. And no, I'm not making any of this up. Headache, abdominal pain, diarrhea, generalized pain, nausea, urinary tract infection, dizziness, vomiting, rash, constipation, flatulence, cough, back pain, weakness, fatigue, malaise, acid regurgitation, allergic reactions, fever, abdominal swelling, abnormally rapid heartbeat, abnormally slow heartbeat, elevated blood pressure, edema, anorexia, irritable colon, esophagus infection, mucosal atrophy of the tongue, dry mouth, dry skin, polyps and/or tumors in the gastrointestinal tract, jaundice, hepatitis, overt liver disease, hypoglycemia, weight gain, deficiency of sodium in the blood, muscle cramps, muscle pain, muscle weakness, joint pain, leg pain, throat pain, psychic disturbances, depression, aggression, hallucinations, confusion, insomnia, nervousness, tremors, apathy, drowsiness, anxiety, dream abnormalities, vertigo, burning, prickling or creepy-crawly feeling on skin, itchy skin, bleeding or hemorrhaging of the nose, severe, painful lesions of the skin or in the mouth, discoloration of skin, inflammation of skin, excessive perspiration, taste perversions, ringing in the ears, frequent urination, pus in the urine, excess sugar in the urine, protein in the urine, blood in the urine, depression of all cellular elements of the blood, decrease of platelets in the blood, weakness of leukocytes in the immune system and anemia. *Yikes!*

Now, before you start to shake your head in disbelief, there's more. There are three side effects that affect only men. Hey guys, you're going to love this: hair loss, development of breasts and, my favorite, testicle pain. And as any man will tell you, he would much prefer painful testicles than some heartburn. Hold on a minute, that's still not all. Heartburn is an unpleasant discomfort in the chest area. Of course, it's nothing like angina, the most crushing, devastating chest pain imaginable. Anyone who has ever endured the unbearable pain of angina shudders at the prospect of ever experiencing it again. You know what I'm getting at, don't you? That's right, the little purple pill for heartburn can cause angina! Wouldn't that be akin to trading a mosquito bite for a shark bite? Who in their right mind would do that? And pay money for the opportunity?

I'd truly like to tell you that that's the end of the list, but it's not. Not by a long shot. Even though you've seen the list of dozens and dozens of side effects, some of which are frightening and brutal, I've yet to tell you the worst of it. I know, can you believe it? Mr. Ripley himself would have trouble with this stranger-than-fiction tale.

*W*hy shouldn't truth be stranger
than fiction? Fiction, after all,
has to make sense.

—MARK TWAIN

So it turns out that the pretty little purple pill *kills*. And not from one side effect, but from *five* different ones. They are listed in the "adverse reaction" section as follows: (1) pancreatitis (some fatal); (2) liver necrosis (some fatal); (3) liver failure (some fatal); (4) severe toxic skin reaction (some fatal); and (5) lesions of throat, skin and gastro-intestinal tract (some fatal).

Since "some" is plural, that means at the very least, two, perhaps more, but at least two deaths for each of the five causes listed. Add 'em up. That's at least ten deaths. Are *you* willing to *die* for your heartburn? When I first read that people actually died, I was interested to know how many hundreds of thousands of people were in the clinical trials. Was it 200,000 or 400,000 or more? The grand total of subjects, both domestic and international, was a whopping 3,096 subjects. How fast would you run to your doctor for the pretty little purple pill if at the end of the ads with all the dancing and blue skies, you heard, "Oh yes, and it can kill you." Obviously, the more Prilosec you take, the more likely you are to die. And the little purple pill is to be taken *every day*. In fact, in the letter accompanying the brochure it states, "Just because you're feeling better doesn't mean you should skip any days. Skipping days could cause your symptoms to return." Too bad they chose not to tell that it could also cause you to meet the grim reaper. So I guess you should take it every day until you either get better or have an adverse drug event, whichever comes first.

Whenever pharmaceutical companies are confronted with the fact that their product(s) can cause some great harm, or death, they all start to sing their favorite, most reliable refrain. It goes something like this: "Oh, that hardly ever happens. It's an extremely rare event. You're more likely to be hit by lightning." Let me ask you a question. If a loved one—your wife or husband, mother or father, or son or daughter—took the little purple pill for heartburn for a few weeks and then dropped dead before your eyes, would your grief be washed away upon learning that it probably wouldn't happen to anyone else for a really long time? Heck no, it wouldn't. When it's *your* loved one being lowered into the ground, statistics don't mean a darn thing, do they?

In the year 2000, enough people were convinced to take Prilosec that the tidy little sum of $6 billion was generated.[1] It did *so* well that the makers of this little gem decided to parlay the success into even greater heights (or depths) with the sequel: Nexium, the little purple pill's big brother. Again, the ads were incessant, and again I sent for the promotional material. When it arrived, I immediately turned to the "adverse reactions," hoping beyond hope that the list of possible side effects would be lower. I whipped out my trusty magnifying glass only to find out that the number of side effects jumped from 80 to 147!

If each year, along with the Oscar, the Grammy, the Emmy, the Tony and others, there was an award given for the most effective and profitable cashectomy, it would be called the "Cashie." The prize would be an eighteen-inch-high, solid-gold dollar sign, and the pharmaceutical industry would win hands-down.

Billions upon billions of dollars are spent every year on drugs to quell the pain that results from doing something as normal, natural and fundamental to life as eating. And every last one of the drugs, either prescription or over-the-counter, is designed to fight the symptoms, not the cause. That way the billions spent this year will be spent again next year and the year after that. The pharmaceutical industry would never in a million years tell you about Live Plant Enzymes, which prevent the problems before they occur and are a mere fraction of the cost.

When I first started taking Live Plant Enzymes regularly in 1995, it wasn't because I was suffering from any kind of pain. I had already figured out how to avoid pain by eating differently. I took them because of the life-extending value of not having to use up my metabolic enzymes on digestion. But as years went by, many of the people I had recommended them to, for the same reason of conserving their metabolic enzymes, started to report back that digestive problems they suffered with for years had disappeared after regularly taking Live Plant Enzymes with their cooked meals.

The words *miracle, godsend* and *lifesaver* have been used more times than I can recall. One acquaintance of mine told me that although he loved pizza, the pain in his stomach was so severe any time he ate it that he stopped eating it altogether. Based on what he had heard from me and others who swore by Live Plant Enzymes, he decided to give it another try. He had two slices of pizza and waited, with antacids in hand, for the pain that he "knew" would come. It never did. The guy was so happy you would think he had won the mega-lottery.

I don't want to give the impression that by taking Live Plant Enzymes all digestive disorders will fall by the wayside. Too many variables exist to make that kind of guarantee. But they can help millions of people, and of that I am certain. And even if they wouldn't help everyone with digestive disorders, the fact that they conserve metabolic enzymes is reason enough to use them. In either event, I would give them a try before swallowing something that could kill me.

I made it my business to find out where to obtain the finest, purest, most reliably high-quality Live Plant Enzymes in the world. It turns out they are produced in Japan, and they are the only ones I now use. In a moment I will tell you how you can obtain the very same ones.

You may presently be taking digestive enzymes that are on the market. There is no comparison. Commercially made enzymes produced from papaya or pineapple fall far short in two very significant ways. First, they are primarily designed to help in digesting proteins, and they only minimally help with fat and starches. Live Plant Enzymes digest all three. Second is the potency issue. Store-bought enzymes are sold by weight in milligrams so you don't actually know what you're getting. They can have fillers, additives, corn starch or any number of other ingredients. The actual amount of enzyme could be minuscule. Plus the caps are usually made of gelatin from steer or horse hooves. Live Plant Enzymes are sold by what is called units of activity. No fillers, no additives; nothing but pure enzyme—with a potency far, far in excess of those sold off the shelf in health-food stores. What you are getting is all enzyme and nothing else, which is why the capsules, which are vegetable-based, are so small.

Since 1995, I have not had a single bite of cooked food without first taking Live Plant Enzymes. And I never will. I take them with me to restaurants and when I travel. If I should forget them (which I rarely ever do), I simply eat only fruit and salad. Quite frankly, I would no more eat cooked food without first taking my Live Plant Enzymes than I would set my foot on a railroad track and let a train run over it just to see how it felt.

I feel that it is my obligation and I would be remiss if I did not urge you to give Live Plant Enzymes a try. Call toll free 1-877-942-4492 or 1-877-215-1212, and you, too, can start to take advantage of one of the great discoveries of our time. You can also contact us online:

Web site: *www.fitforlifetime.com*
e-mail: *info@fitforlifetime.com*

While on this subject, you should know that several pure enzyme products are available which address and improve a wide array of different physical conditions. I am compelled to briefly tell you of two of these products, based on a recently released report from a comprehensive government study.

As I'm sure you already know, cardiovascular disease

(conditions related to the heart and bloodstream) is the number-one killer of Americans. In fact, cardiovascular disease kills more people than all other diseases **combined**. High blood pressure (hypertension) is a major cause of all heart attacks and strokes, and according to the above-referenced study, high blood pressure is once again on the rise, after a decades-long downward trend.

According to one of the authors of the recent government study, "The jump coincides with a sharp increase in the number of Americans who are overweight or obese, a major cause of hypertension."[2]

The two enzyme products to which I refer are CardioZyme and RenewZyme.

CardioZyme contains the newly discovered enzyme nattokinase, along with six additional enzymes and a blend of minerals known to support *nattokinase*. It was first discovered by a doctor in Japan and has been shown to support and assist the only enzyme in the body that removes blood clots. Its ability to break down the protein structure of the clot is what has generated such excitement about its discovery, since no other "nonsynthetic" enzyme has the ability to do this as efficiently. In the past, pharmaceutical drugs have been administered intravenously for this same purpose immediately following a heart attack or stroke to prevent further risk and damage.

RenewZyme is a high-potency blend of proteolytic enzymes (enzymes that break down proteins) intended to support circulation, reduce inflammation and speed healing. The enzyme bromelain, in particular, is known for its ability to reduce the symptoms of inflammation, as a result of its becoming active at just above normal human body temperature. Bromelain, along with other enzymes, seems to be drawn to the site of the inflammation, and once there, these combined enzymes help reduce inflammation by breaking down the proteins that restrict blood flow and impede healing.

On page 239, you will find toll-free numbers and a Web site, both of which will provide information about these enzyme products.

CHAPTER TEN

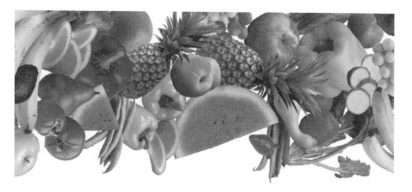

QUESTIONS ANYONE?

With health everything is a source
of pleasure; without it nothing else, whatever
it may be, is enjoyable. Health is by far
the most important element
in human happiness.

—ARTHUR SCHOPENHAUER

There's no way for me to address every possible question that may arise as a result of reading a book such as this, so I'm not going to try. But more than three decades of being asked questions is enough for me to know what the most common questions are. Following are the ten most frequently asked questions from the last thirty-plus years.

1. **What about protein? Will I get enough if I start eating more living food and less cooked food?**

    Without a doubt this is the one question asked more often than any other. It reflects how supremely effective the animal-products industry has been in its quest to bamboozle, deceive and mislead a confused public. In every book I've ever written, I have discussed the subject of protein. Opinions on how much should be eaten and from what source vary as far as the pendulum can swing—everything from eat only protein and nothing else to don't eat any at all. Studies abound proving both extremes and everything in between. In *Fit for Life II*, I utilized numerous scientific studies, more than a hundred, to prove my basic approach, which is: The less you eat, the better. But I can assure you that there is someone somewhere who can produce studies that prove that the *more* you eat, the better. I'm tired of playing the game of dueling studies; it does nothing but confuse an already confused public. With the proper funding, you can prove anything. I'm not going to ignore completely scientific studies, because there are some that are so impressive that no one can fault them, but for this discussion I'm going to rely most heavily on the most trustworthy tools we human beings have: our common sense, instincts and sense of logic, the greatest enemies of the overeducated mind.

Before getting into it, I want to make it clear that I am *not* a vegetarian. I have no vested interest either way. My only concern is what's the healthiest. I was a vegetarian for over a quarter of a century, but hey, things change. I've always told my readers that if they crave something for a long time, it must be something the body wants or needs, so have it and see how you feel. One day out of the clear blue sky, after not having meat for twenty-five years, I started to crave a charbroiled steak the way a lion craves a wildebeest. I couldn't get it out of my head no matter how much I tried to ignore the craving or convince myself that it was some kind of aberrant desire. So finally I decided to eat the steak, throw it up and move on. The only thing was, I enjoyed it, and I felt great. Of course, I had it with salad and vegetables. Now about twice a week I have some kind of animal product like steak, salmon or chicken—whatever I want. I definitely don't have it every day or even two days in a row, and I always have a salad as an accompaniment. You know, the healthy way.

I haven't changed my mind about vegetarianism being the healthiest way to go—I'm convinced it is—but as stated, understanding and accepting something intellectually is one thing; doing it is another.

Here's something to ponder: How did we humans make it before we started eating meat? If eating protein is so crucial to health, as some proponents claim, how did we make it for the thousands, hundreds of thousands, or millions of years—or however long it was that we roamed the Earth before we discovered fire and started charbroiling our four-legged friends? Somehow we managed to survive on fruits, berries, nuts, seeds, tubers, grasses and vegetables well enough to continue the species. How?

When you think of a true carnivore on the land or in the air or sea, what do you think of? A lion, an eagle, a shark? What particular features do these animals all possess that we humans do not? Built-in tools for capture, killing and devouring, right? Speed, strength, claws, teeth and talons. These are tools true animal eaters are born with. We don't have them. If you were somehow abandoned or marooned somewhere with nothing but your own hide, no guns or knives, no cook stove or fire, nothing but your own wits, what would you seek out to eat? Would you try chasing down an antelope or wild boar? Even if you somehow caught up with it, what would you do then? Even if you managed to overcome one with a rock or something, what then? Are you going to tear it open somehow and dig in? Eating the flesh and blood raw, the way any other self-respecting carnivore would? Maybe you would do this with something smaller like a rabbit or a squirrel. The only thing is, they're far more adept at getting away from you than you are at catching them.

Do you salivate with anticipation at the thought of scarfing down the entrails of a dead animal? True meat-eaters do. In fact, if you didn't have the convenience of going to the grocery store for a neatly packaged cut of beef, would you look forward to slaughtering a steer and obtaining what you want for yourself? Would you slog through the guts and gore and look forward to doing the same the next day and the day after that? If you think I'm being disgusting, that helps make my point. It is not in your nature to do these things. If you were hungry to the point of starving, and you were chasing some animal with the hopes of catching it and somehow ultimately getting it into your stomach, and the animal, with you hot on its tail, ran through an apple orchard, what would you do? Continue to chase the animal or stuff yourself with apples? Your hands are not designed for tearing into the bellies of animals. They are, however, perfectly designed for picking the fruit from trees.

While we're on the subject of animals, what animal do you think of as the strongest of all? What animals have been used for centuries because of their strength and endurance? The ones that can lift heavy loads or plow fields for hours on end without tiring. Elephants, oxen, water buffalo, camels, horses, mules. All of these, indeed the most powerful animals on Earth, eat only plant foods. Strict carnivores sleep over twenty hours a day. That's why you won't ever see a tiger pulling a plow. An African water buffalo can weigh nearly a ton. They ripple with muscles, are incredibly strong and strike fear into anyone or anything in their path when on a full-out charge. A bull elephant can weigh more than ten tons, carry astounding loads and pull trees out of the ground. They live on grass and leaves.

Did you ever see the movie *Gorillas in the Mist*? It was about the silverback gorilla. These impressive beasts are three times the size of a man but thirty times as strong. Their muscle development is astounding. They eat bamboo leaves and fruit. Think you could arm-wrestle a gorilla and win?

How do all these animals develop such imposing muscular strength without ever eating protein? Ever wonder about that? We love eating cows for protein, and it's supposed to be the ideal protein for us. Ever see a cow eating a steak? What does a cow eat to produce all that protein? Grass and grains.

So what's the answer? Obviously, all animals, including human beings, need protein to live, there's no doubt about that. The same way elephants and water buffalos and gorillas obtain their protein is the way we humans can obtain ours. Protein is built from amino acids. That's it, plain and simple. Amino acids build protein and are resplendent in the plant kingdom. That's why an elephant or a gorilla has no protein deficiencies. They obtain all the amino acids they need from the source—the plant kingdom.

When you eat a piece of chicken, that's exactly what it is: chicken protein. By putting it into your body, it doesn't magically turn into human protein. No more so than if you ate an animal's liver would it go into your body and become part of *your* liver. An amino acid chain can have from 50 to 100,000 amino acids. They must be broken down, reassembled and built into human protein. You can get amino acids from meat, but we don't eat meat raw, and the heating of amino acids destroys many of them and causes others to coagulate so the amino acid availability is extremely poor. Amino acids are delicate and affected by heat the same way other nutrients and enzymes are. When a lion eats a zebra, the amino acids from the zebra are broken down and reassembled into lion protein. Fortunately for the lion, it is too stupid to figure out how to cook the zebra before eating it, so the amino acids remain intact.

Ever notice that carnivorous animals don't ever eat other carnivorous animals except under the most extreme circumstances? Why do you think meat-eating animals eat plant-eating animals? Plants can manufacture amino acids from air, soil and water; animals can't. They either have to eat the plant directly for their amino acids or obtain them indirectly by eating an animal that has eaten the plant. Meat-eating animals instinctively eat animals that have eaten plants. And no matter which they eat, the plant or the animal, both are raw—no cooking.

> **O**ften the less there is to justify
> a traditional custom, the harder
> it is to get rid of it.
>
> —Mark Twain

Over the years, people have been thoroughly conditioned to automatically think of some kind of meat when the subject of protein comes up. The conditioning has been relentless and successful. It's almost comical to even suggest that someone would think of a fruit or vegetable salad for protein over a steak or a hamburger. But I'll tell you what, the amino acids in a salad are a lot more available and easily utilizable than the amino acids in meat that have been deranged by heat. It may take you a while to overcome the conditioning, but if you are looking for high-quality protein, which is the same as saying high-quality amino acids, the finest and best source comes from living food, not cooked food. Remember Pottenger's cats? They were fed only protein foods, either cooked or uncooked. The cats on uncooked protein thrived, while the health of the cats on cooked protein suffered.

Here's an interesting tidbit on the subject of amino acids and their protein-building capabilities. In 1914, studies were conducted to see if rats fared better on the amino acids from animals or from plants.[1] Since a rat's metabolism and requirements for protein are diametrically different from those of human beings, rats fared better on the protein from animals. So the results of the studies proclaimed that protein from animals is superior to protein from plants—for humans! That's what the animal-products industry ran with, even though it was subsequently shown that those studies, which were not conducted on humans, were therefore inapplicable to humans. The myth was ignited, and it still burns today.

Here's yet one last tidbit on the subject. I told you there are some studies that are so impeccably conducted and reliable that they are acknowledged as useful by nearly everyone. Such a study is the China Health Project,[2] an extensive study done with the help of researchers at Cornell University, Oxford University and the Chinese government. This extraordinary, long-term study has been hailed as "one of the most rigorous and conclusive studies in the history of health research."[3] Books have been written on the mountain of data collected from this one study, and I want to tell you two of the findings. The first has to do with what are referred to as the "diseases of affluence": heart disease, cancer, diabetes, osteoporosis and obesity.

In the United States the diseases of affluence are rampant. In China, they are either practically non-existent or notably uncommon. The China Health Project pointed out that one of the most significant reasons for this difference is the fact that the Chinese people obtain 7 percent of their protein from animal products while Americans obtain 70 percent of their protein from animal products. Ten times as much! Second, as regards obesity, which is rare in China, the Chinese people eat 20 percent more calories than Americans, but Americans are 25 percent fatter.

The animal-products industry makes its living selling its products the same way any other industry with a product makes its living. They want you to buy what they're selling. They spend hundreds of millions of dollars to convince you to eat what they're selling for your protein needs. It's business. I don't know if reading a few paragraphs is going to overcome decades of propaganda and conditioning—maybe it will, maybe it won't. In either event, every once in a while eat a couple of bananas for your protein (amino acids). You know, like the *Gorillas in the Mist*.

2. **If I were to decrease my consumption of dairy products, what would be the best way to make up for the lost calcium?**

The snow job put over on the American public continues. Back in the chapter on fruit, I was answering the question that interviewers so frequently ask: "What is the very best and very worst food we can put into our bodies?" I made it abundantly clear that the very best was fruit and said I would get to the very worst later. Well, here we are. If the people of the United States were to somehow become aware of the true and actual effect that dairy products have had on health, they would be lined up to sue the same way they're lined up to sue the tobacco industry.

We know a lot about nutrition, and there's far more to learn. I don't claim to have an answer to every question or to understand every nuance of what is or is not good for the body, but I am as equally certain of the harmfulness of dairy products as I am of fruit's value. There is not a malady of the human body, serious or minor, that dairy products don't contribute to, cause or worsen.

As with my answer to the protein question, I'm not going to load you up with hundreds of scientific studies to make my point. I did that in *Fit for Life II*. I'll use some, but I would rather appeal once again to your common sense, instinct and sense of logic. The multibillion-dollar dairy industry is in business to make money, and no tactic, honest or underhanded, is off-limits. I don't begrudge the making of money. I want to make money also; everyone has to pay the rent. But I'd like to come by my money through performing some kind of beneficial service or providing a healthful product, not by way of the cashectomy.

There can be no more effective selling tool for an industry than convincing people that they will suffer and become ill without using their product. And that is exactly what the dairy industry has done—quite ingeniously, I might add. After all, every health expert, no matter what discipline is practiced, acknowledges that a diet high in fiber and low in fat and cholesterol is best. Dairy products are extremely *high* in fat and cholesterol, and are *devoid* of fiber—the absolute, polar opposite of what is being recommended by one and all.

So how do you get people to feel they can't live without this product that actually has nothing to offer, unless you like having a stuffed-up nose? *That* was the task. Calcium! If people could be frightened into thinking that their bones would become brittle like dried-out kindling unless they consumed dairy products for the calcium, the dairy industry would be home-free. Has their ploy worked? What's the first thing that pops into your mind when you hear the word "calcium"? Women in particular have been preyed upon by this scheme by holding the threat of osteoporosis over their heads like a guillotine.

Here's the question I would like for you to ponder: Is it possible Mother Nature, the Grand Creator, God, the intelligence of the universe that created us and everything else in existence, would somehow forget to make something as crucial to life as calcium available to us, thereby forcing us to become the one and only species of mammal the length and breadth of the planet to *never* be weaned? Shall we never be weaned? C'mon now, how could we fall for such a preposterous suggestion? In the grand scheme of things, every mammal on Earth—whether it's a dog, a cat, a whale, a cow, a rhinoceros, a giraffe, a wolf or a human being, large or small, ferocious or docile—shall have as its first food a highly nutritious milk that flows from its mother's breast. Each species has its own milk that is unique to that species and no other. It is designed specifically to be the first and only food to supply the newborn with the best possible food during infancy, and every mammal, whether elephant or mouse, *stops* drinking milk once it is weaned, never to have milk again—not its own mother's milk nor the milk of another species. Do you actually think that this supremely intelligent plan, designed and implemented by the Grand Creator, applies to every species of mammal in existence except *us?* There is not another instance in nature where an animal, once weaned, will continue to suckle or start to suckle later in life. It does not *ever* happen.

My illness is due to
my doctor's insistence that I drink
milk, a whitish fluid they force
down helpless babies.

—W. C. FIELDS

Not only have we humans figured out a way to disregard and defy the awesome design of life itself, but look at the animal we turn to in order to do so. Even if we were somehow able to continue drinking the milk of our own species, it would still be wrong— milk is for infants, not grown-ups. But we don't go to an animal that is even remotely close to us in size, like a chimpanzee. In fact, most people might recoil or be offended at the very idea of drinking chimpanzee milk. Yet we have somehow been psychologically manipulated into accepting as reasonable the drinking of cow's milk. How about milk from a dog, or a horse, or a hyena or a sheep? Would you drink those? Why not? The only reason people are accustomed to cow's milk is because they were trained to drink it from childhood. It could just as easily have been hog milk that we were made to accept as normal, in which case we would very likely be offended by the idea of drinking cow's milk.

Cow's milk, being uniquely constituted for its young, is the food for a ninety-pound calf at birth, which will ultimately reach the weight of somewhere between 1,000 and 2,000 pounds in only two years. Human milk, being uniquely constituted and suited for its young, is the food for a five- to ten-pound infant who will ultimately reach the weight of somewhere between 100 and 200 pounds in eighteen years. In other words, cow's milk is specifically designed for an animal that will grow very large, very fast. Do you think that's something people who are trying to lose weight want? To get real big, real fast, like a cow? Plus, is milk (or products made from milk like cheese, yogurt, ice cream, etc.) consumed in its natural state? No, it's pasteurized, which means that it's heated to a temperature so high that nothing living could survive. Everything good you're hoping to get from it is either destroyed or deranged.

The protein component in milk is a thick, coarse substance called casein. It is broken down in the body by the enzyme rennin. Because Nature's intent is for us to be weaned from milk and not have it again, by age three or four rennin is nonexistent in the human digestive tract in all but a very small number of people. The idea that the dairy industry would have us believe that we should consume dairy products to get calcium is absolutely preposterous. The calcium in cow's milk is, first of all, much coarser than the calcium in human's milk, and second, the calcium in cow's milk is bound to the casein, which prevents it from being absorbed by the human body. There is 300 percent more casein in cow's milk than there is in human milk, and it is used to make one of the strongest wood glues in existence. Sounds like just the thing to eat for successful weight loss, doesn't it? Glue!

The big issue in all of this is, of course, calcium and osteoporosis. The human skeleton is a thing of beauty. We are born with 350 or so bones, which fuse into the approximately 206 bones in an adult skeleton. Through the loss of calcium, bones can become so porous that they can break with very little provocation. Going over a bump in the road while driving, sneezing or even being hugged can cause fractures. High-protein, high-acid diets cause calcium to be leached from the bones. There is irrefutable evidence to prove this, more than you could read in a lifetime. Proponents of diets high in meat and dairy products will try to deny it, but it's like trying to deny the sun is hot. It is an indefensible position. Meat and dairy contribute more to osteoporosis than any other factor.[4] The Masai of Africa, Inuits and Greenlanders eat enormously high-protein diets, almost to the exclusion of all else. They develop osteoporosis at a very early age and are bent, disabled and decrepit in their twenties and thirties.[5] On the other hand, the Abkhazians of Russia, the Vilcabambans of Ecuador and the Hunzas eat a diet that minimizes protein food, and they stand erect with little or no osteoporosis well into their eighties and nineties.[6]

The dairy industry would have you believe that dairy products would put an end to the problem of osteoporosis. This is ironic in light of the fact that dairy products *cause* osteoporosis. I can understand the dairy industry's trying to do whatever it can to sell more product. What I find objectionable, in fact criminal, are the so-called "experts," the medical doctors, dieticians and nutritionists who should know better, but have failed to educate themselves, who are out there telling an unsuspecting public to consume dairy products for calcium. It would be like telling an alcoholic to sober up on a bottle of whiskey.

Consider this: The four countries of the world whose population consume the greatest amount of dairy products are the United States, Great Britain, Sweden and Finland.[7] The four countries of the world whose population has the highest incidence of osteoporosis are the United States, Great Britain, Sweden and Finland.[8] The countries whose population consumes the least of amount of dairy products are the African and Asian countries. The countries whose population suffers the least incidence of osteoporosis are the

African and Asian countries.[9] Exactly what else do you need to know that will convince you?

Just in case you're not convinced (and I can hardly believe that anyone isn't), here's the clincher: I told you about the China Health Project, the study considered to be so impeccably conducted and well-respected. There are approximately 290 million people in the United States. There are a billion *more* people in China, making it the largest population on Earth by far. The Chinese people don't like dairy products. They find them foul-smelling and -tasting, and they don't partake. Osteoporosis is so rare in China that there is not even a word for it in the Chinese language. Another noted scientist at the National Institutes of Health points out that, "The Chinese consume no cow's milk or dairy products, yet they have among the lowest rates of osteoporosis in the world."[10] And all the hired celebrities with milk mustaches are not going to change that.

The truth is more important
than the facts.

—Frank Lloyd Wright

Here's the question I would like for you to ask yourself: If it is true that cow's milk contains so much high-quality calcium, where does it come from? Cows don't drink milk. They don't take supplements. Where are they getting all the calcium? From the exact same place they're getting all the amino acids they need to build their perfect protein. And you know where that is, don't you? All together now, one, two, three—*from plants!* Just like the Chinese people who have no osteoporosis. Everything that grows out of the ground has calcium in it. Everything. What you should bear in mind is that your calcium intake is only one-half of the story. The other half is the loss of calcium that is used to neutralize the acid of a cooked diet, especially highly acidic animal products, meat and dairy. When you commit to increasing the amount of living food you are eating to 50 percent and decreasing the amount of cooked food you are eating to 50 percent, you are eating a diet that raises the level of calcium intake while lowering the level of foods that cause calcium loss. Now there's a combination that's hard to beat.

I want to share a little personal item with you. I have thoroughly documented the excruciating stomachaches that plagued my youth. When I was a little boy, my bedtime was 8:00 P.M. Generally, kids don't want to go to bed when they're told to, so all manner of ruses are concocted to stay up a bit later. With me, as far back as I can remember, when I heard, "Okay, Harvey, bedtime," I had this ritual that I went through. I'd say, "Can I have a glass of milk first?" Of course, thinking it was a healthy thing to do, my mom always let me have it, frequently with cookies. I was able to squeeze out another ten to fifteen minutes before going to bed. Every night, I would go to sleep with a belly full of acid that took its toll. So very many nights, I would wake up in pain, sit down with my pillow on my lap and try to sleep that way. For some reason, I was convinced that sitting doubled-over would make the stomachache go away. I would awaken in the morning and guess what was the first thing I did? I had a big glass of pasteurized orange juice. Another dose of acid. For years, every night the last thing I had was a glass of acid, and every morning the first thing I had was a glass of acid. How sad that it never dawned on anyone that my "delicate stomach" was the result of my dietary habits. Of course in those days, people who attributed health problems to diet were classified as kooks. Medical doctors considered the study of nutrition to be a waste of time.

Rarely does a day go by that I don't thank the powers that be who saw fit to extricate me from the darkness and shine the light of understanding into my life so I can live without pain. I know that there are those of you, whether you agree with what you have read here about the dairy/calcium connection or not, who are going to want to take some type of calcium supplements, even if it's just for peace of mind. I have no problem with this, so long as it's a super-high-quality, organic, properly balanced calcium. I have located such a product, and it is the only one I would recommend. You can read all about it in appendix I.

3. **As a mother of young children, obviously I want to do the best I can for them. Is this way of eating safe and healthy for children?**

Goodness gracious, yes! *All* living bodies, young and old, need living food. And given some of the dire statistics now attributed to children, never in history has the need been greater for our young. It was in the late 1950s or early 1960s that McDonald's foisted the fast-food mentality onto our culture, and children's health has headed downhill ever since. Perhaps you recall the opening line in the introduction of this book. The picture of that overweight kid on the cover of *Newsweek* magazine was one of the reasons I decided to write this book in the first place.

I realize that I have called to your attention several times the unprecedented problem of obesity in children today. As one more piece of evidence to support that fact, consider that drastic stomach bypass surgery for obesity, which is performed on some 100,000 adults a year, is now emerging as a viable option for some of the 15 percent of youngsters in the United States who are severely overweight or obese.[11] This surgery is performed on children in spite of the fact that the long-term side effects are completely unknown. One can only imagine what kind of nutritional deficiencies will occur in these children at a time in their lives when their bodies have an urgent need for nutrients in order to keep growing. Never in all of history has the need to teach children about the importance of living food been greater.

Mankind owes to the child
the best it has to give.

—United Nations Declaration

There is no circumstance in life where living food would not be beneficial. Whether a person is young or old, in poor health or good health, living food is always welcomed by the body and put to good use. But if there *is* a time when it is particularly important, or should I say a time when there is an extra incentive to eat living food, it would have to be during childhood. During those formative years, children are developing the likes, dislikes and habits that will be the foundation for the way they eat as adults, or perhaps the rest of their lives. That is why it saddens me deeply to say that there are millions of children who have *never* in their entire lives eaten a single living meal, not once, not ever, unless, of course, they were fortunate enough to have been breast-fed.

The way marketers and advertisers have convinced parents to feed their children seems like a plot to destroy their health before they even have a chance at life. It is impossible to talk about children and the marketing of products to or for children without also revisiting the subject of cashectomies. You should know that a successful cashectomy is no respecter of age. Even infants, the most innocent and helpless of all, are sacrificed on the altar of profits. How? Baby formulas.

That's right, you read it correctly. Once again, I must bring up the incomprehensible intelligence that rules and directs every activity of the cosmos in which we live, with a perfection we cannot even begin to grasp. What else but this intelligence could possibly come up with such a perfect plan for the feeding of newborns? But there's no money to be made in women breast-feeding. After all, milk flows for free, for two years or more. And don't think it wasn't a seemingly insurmountable challenge to somehow convince women that breast milk, the food God makes for infants, could somehow be equaled, even surpassed by some concoction brewed up in a laboratory.

Have they succeeded? Today infant formulas are a multibillion-dollar concern. Nature's simple but elegant plan for the newborn is milk that is highly nutritious, perfectly balanced with all the nutrients necessary to support life, naturally sweet, the perfect temperature, and *free* as part of the gift of life. Plus, and this is of immeasurable importance, the first substance to flow from a mother's breast, prior to the flow of milk, is a yellowish fluid called colostrum. This substance coats the infant's digestive tract and plays a crucial role in the development of its immune system for the remainder of the child's life.

The cashectomist's version is a vile concoction of synthesized chemicals, haphazardly thrown together in a laboratory, sweetened with processed, refined sugar and heated to a temperature so high *no* living thing could possibly survive, let alone the delicate nutrients required by the newborn. Plus, it has no colostrum. Notwithstanding what you have been led to believe by poorly educated, hired doctors, formulas are, one and all, mucous-forming, disease-producing swill, and are hugely responsible for the ear infections, colic, rashes and other disturbances that plague the early years of most babies who are not breast-fed. And you are tricked into paying good money for this rank impostor.

In over thirty years of study, I have never, *ever* known of even one child with an ear infection who was not fed formula, cow's milk or both. *Not one!* And as soon as they are removed from the child's diet, ear infections "miraculously" disappear. Every year over 30,000 children under the age of five die of respiratory disease syndrome. That's more than eighty children dying every day. The journal *Lancet* identifies the substance "muco-protein" in the lungs of these young, dead children.[12] Now where do you think this "muco-protein" comes from?

By the way, did you know that when formulas were introduced, in order to get things rolling, women were actually convinced to have shots immediately after giving birth that dried up their milk so there was no alternative to formula? These women were told by their physicians that formula, in addition to being more convenient, was just as good as breast milk. Since they were told this by their trusted doctors, they had the shots that dried up their milk and put their babies on formula. And that, dear friends, is a first-rate cashectomy.

> The truth which makes us free is
> for the most part the truth
> we prefer not to hear.
>
> —HERBERT AGAR

Once kids are off the formula bottle, they are led like sheep directly to breakfast cereals and the fast-food chains. Marketers know there are billions of dollars to be made advertising products to entice children who are highly impressionable and easily persuaded. The average child sees 10,000 food commercials on TV a year.[13] Children don't make their food choices based on what is healthy and good for them. Advertisers play to them with toys, games, snappy jingles, happy clowns, dancing animals, action figures, cartoon characters, anything that can get them to harangue their parents into getting them what they want. The next time you're in the grocery store, make note of what section is one of the largest in the store, with the most shelf-space. Breakfast cereals. These dreadful boxes of offal, without a single, solitary saving grace, are passed off as good food for your child. The number-one ingredient in all of them is refined sugar. They are doused in a chemical bath of preservatives, additives, colored dyes, hydrogenated oils and other multisyllablic words that you can't even pronounce, let alone know the meaning of, such as butylated hydroxytoluene (BHT), which will prevent the hydrogenated vegetable oil from going rancid. They are heated at a temperature so high that nothing of nutritional value could survive. They are processed, refined and entirely destroyed—killed.

Pick up a box of one of Kelloggs's new and innovative boxes designed to snare children, such as one in the Disney collection. What kid can resist Mickey Mouse grinning at him or her? Or a box of Post Fruity Pebbles, where they try to associate what's in the box with something truly natural and nutritious like fruit by putting pictures of fruit on the front and a game on the back that says, "Welcome to Fruitrageous Fun Park." There is nothing even remotely associated with fruit in the box except the imitation chemical colorings. A box of General Mills' Lucky Charms has a special note on the side from the American Heart Association announcing that the cereal has no cholesterol in it. After you wade through all the games, puzzles, whistles, toys and other free prizes, read the ingredients. It's frightening. You'll find a veritable riot of chemicals sweetened by all manner of different processed sugars and colored with red dyes #3 and #40, yellow dyes #5 and #6, and blue dyes #1 and #2. (Yellow dye #5 has been shown to be particularly damaging to children and associated with behavioral problems. Red dye #40, the most widely used dye, has been acknowledged by the FDA as causing these same types of adverse behavioral reactions in children.)[14]

And into this worthless, disease-producing slag is squirted some synthesized, inorganic, chemical vitamins so the manufacturer can put on the box, "Now fortified with essential vitamins." They in no way serve the same function as do the vitamins in living food. The scheme is to trick you into thinking the addition of some synthetic nutrient miraculously transforms an adulterated, denatured, overly processed mixture of dead food and chemicals into something of value for your child. This stuff isn't food; it's an insult to life. Oh, I almost forgot, what's poured over this concoction? Milk!

Let advertisers spend the same amount of money improving their product that they do on advertising and they wouldn't have to advertise it.

—WILL ROGERS

Let me show you how kids can go through an entire day without even a hint of living food. Upon awakening in the morning, perhaps to start the day off right, they are given a glass of orange juice. Only thing is, it's pasteurized. Then onto one of the bowls of sweetened chemicals described above with some mucous-forming milk. Maybe a piece of toasted white bread or a Pop-Tart. Off to school. When lunch is served, it's hot dogs, hamburgers, pizza, sloppy Joes, chips, French fries, Jell-O and milk or soda. Maybe, *maybe* an apple, probably not. Later for a snack, a candy bar or a bag of chips or some cookies. Home for dinner. Macaroni and cheese, beans and franks, or some type of fast food. The only living food the entire day is a slice of tomato or shredded lettuce on their hamburger. Sometimes, for convenience, the child may take to school or have at home a preorganized meal called Oscar Meyer Lunchables. Have you seen these? The entire side panel of the box is the ingredient list. It's like another language. It's amazing this stuff can actually be called food. I can't imagine people reading the full ingredient list, which is frightening *and* challenging, and still giving it to someone they love. All of it is processed, refined, heated and *dead*. Hot dogs, hamburgers, pizza, ham, bologna, cheese, candy, potato chips, soda pop, cookies, cinnamon rolls with icing, and something called "cheddar-cheese food." I don't even want to know what that is. It's as though everything that can be wrong and hurtful for a young growing body is dumped into one of these boxes to be served up to your child. It's all so easy and convenient. I'll tell you something: Convenience should *not* be the number-one priority for the feeding of children.

I'm not saying that this way of feeding children is the norm, not by a long shot. Even though I know there are some people reading this right now who are thinking, "Oh my goodness, he just described the way my kid eats," I also know that parents are doing the best they can for their kids and trying to feed them right. I'm just trying to make a point and show that more effort is required by parents to help their children learn *now* that what they put into their bodies plays an important role in the way they feel. The only place they will learn this is from *you*, not the people who will try any subterfuge, any ploy possible to sell a product even though it may contribute mightily to your children's ill health.

It's no coincidence that we are in the third generation of children being raised on junk food (a generation is twenty years), and children's health is at an all-time low. Obesity, asthma, diabetes, learning disabilities and much more, have all increased to unprecedented numbers. I told you that adults eat approximately 10 percent living food and 90 percent cooked food. It's *worse* for children. They have not been taught to eat living food, and the results are now unavoidably right up in our faces.

You don't need Lieutenant Columbo to figure out that I'm not a big fan of the pharmaceutical industry. It's not that I'm trying to discourage the use of drugs under any circumstances; sometimes in certain situations drugs are unavoidable and that is all there is to it. What I have a problem with is the unnecessary overprescribing of drugs that has become a way of life in the United States. The pharmaceutical industry is the biggest money-making concern ever, with the highest net profit of any industry—more than oil, more than tobacco. In 2000, the pharmaceutical industry took in $125 billion.[15] In 2001 it jumped to $142 billion,[16] and one government agency says by 2008 it will be at $243 billion.[17] Here we are awash in drugs, and it is going to *increase* by 70 percent. We're already at eleven drugs for every man, woman and child,[18] and it's projected to jump to over eighteen per person in the United States.

I firmly believe that if the whole material medica, as now used, could be sunk to the bottom of the sea it would be better for mankind and all the worse for the fishes.

—OLIVER WENDELL HOLMES

There is only one possible result of the deplorable eating habits of children: more pain, more ill health and more disease. There's no way around it. And you know what that means, don't you? More drugs! The appalling state of health among children, while a deep concern for most everyone, is a promising window of opportunity for the drug industry. It's a way to expand sales and be sure to reach that goal of $243 billion, which would mean $665 million spent on drugs every day of the year. Not bad since all we spend today is a mere $390 million a day. There's a long way to go, but with the help of an ever-growing population of sick children, there's every hope that the goal can be met.

You must think I'm being awfully cynical, but I'm not making up this stuff. Senior citizens are already drowning in drugs, so where will the new sales come from? I saw an article in the newspaper with the subheadline that read, "Children: Fastest Growing Group of Prescription Drug Users."[19] The article, along with some alarming facts about how much of an increase there has been in the amount of time children spend medicated, stated that, "Use of prescription drugs is growing faster among children than it is among senior citizens and baby boomers, the two traditionally high consumer groups." And there you have it.

Poor eating habits not only affect a child's physical health, but emotional health suffers as well. Their bodies are struggling with the toxins that are circulating in their systems, and their diet simply does not supply enough fuel and nutrients to deal with it. Children under these circumstances will start to become ornery, defiant, obstinate and hyperactive, and they have no idea what's beating them up. They will be diagnosed with attention deficit disorder (ADD) or attention deficit hyperactivity disorder (ADHD) and put on powerful mood-altering drugs. Some 5 million kids have already been diagnosed with these two so-called "learning disabilities."[20] They are prescribed Ritalin, Cylert, Lithium and an array of antidepressants that have horrific side effects. Powerful antidepressants such as Paxil and Zoloft are being prescribed for *kids*. From 1995 to 1996, prescriptions for Prozac for children ages six to twelve increased by an appalling 209 percent![21] All along, they continue to eat the same denatured, devitalized, fast-food-laden diets.

These powerful drugs are administered, and they

haven't even been tested to see if they are safe for children. The vast majority of prescription drugs are developed for adults, not kids. In October 2002, a federal court threw out legislation that would have required drug companies to test adult medications before giving them to children. The Associated Press reported that, "The ruling means that drug companies may continue to sell medicines approved for adults, but often prescribed for children, without studies showing they are safe and effective for kids or to determine appropriate dosages."[22] Kind of warms your heart, doesn't it? And unless the drug makers are forced by legislation to determine if their products are safe for kids, they'll *never* do it on their own. Too expensive. Besides, that money could be put to better use sending out unsolicited free samples to people who never asked for them. As though not enough people are already being prescribed drugs, Eli Lilly came up with an innovative way to increase sales even more. After inappropriately peeking at people's private medical records and finding out which ones showed a history of depression, Lilly sent out a free, one-month trial supply of one of its best sellers, Prozac.[23] No prescription, no problem. One sixteen-year-old boy was sent the drug with a letter congratulating him on being one step closer to full recovery. His parents were not as enthusiastic as Eli Lilly. Ultimately, a lawsuit had to be filed to force Lilly to stop the practice (of course). The lawyer who represented the plaintiffs had a suggestion for drug companies inclined to mail unsolicited samples: "What they should be doing is developing a drug to diminish their greed."

I wonder if you know Maureen Kennedy Salaman. If you don't, you should. She's one of the unsung heroes in all of this. Maureen is the president of the National Health Federation in Monrovia, California. For decades she has been battling it out with the lobbyists and lawmakers, trying to protect you and your children from the unbridled greed and avarice of those who would gladly sacrifice your children's health for their own selfish purposes. In her words, "We are maiming, sickening and addicting our own children in an industrial orgy of chemically altered foods and drugs on a scale so vast as to call into question our collective sanity."[24]

I'm spending time on this subject because it's so very important. There's no price that can be put on teaching a child about proper diet early in life.

Before leaving this subject I want to share something truly interesting that is relevant for both children and grown-ups. Deep in the center of the brain lies its oldest and most primitive region. It's referred to as the limbic brain. The limbic system plays a key role in emotions, and it developed early in evolution. It is involved with the rigidly programmed, instinctive behavior necessary for our survival. Think of the brain as being two brains, the older, primitive brain (limbic) and the newer, higher brain that developed over and around it. The limbic brain is associated with the most basic, urgent and immediate needs: pain and pleasure, fight and flight, attack and defense, reward and punishment, fear, rage and docility, sleep and wakefulness, gathering of food, obtaining shelter. Spontaneous violence, with no regard for consequences or ethical consideration, is an activity of the limbic brain.

The higher (or new) brain, on the other hand, is associated with the more lofty aspects of life: friendship, camaraderie, sharing, nurturing, high aspirations, appreciation of music and art, desire to do good for others. Volunteering to work with disadvantaged children or read to the elderly are activities associated with the higher brain.

An unfortunate aspect of life today is aberrant behavior of some kind—limbic activities. I think of the serial snipers of October 2002 who killed and terrorized so many people. I think of kids who take guns to school and kill their classmates. When I was a kid, we were checked to see if we brought gum to school; today they walk through metal detectors to make sure they don't bring knives and guns. I remember the Columbine shooting and the other rash of shootings of family and friends by children. Everybody had an opinion as to why it was happening. Talk shows were rife with experts pointing the finger of blame at violence in movies and on TV, violent video games, domestic violence, the high rate of divorce among couples with children, violence in sports—all manner of causes were named. And although I'm certain that each of those factors contributed to some degree, I was astonished that not once did I hear anyone attribute this kind of deviant behavior to diet. Everything was attributed to external influences and not one word about what internal influences were being manifested. Here's the punchline to all this. The limbic brain, the one responsible for all the aberrant behavior I'm referring to, requires *one-fifth* the energy that the higher brain requires.[25]

Think about it. Here we are, well into at the very *least* the second generation of kids raised on junk or fast food, and we are faced with an unprecedented amount of what can only be described as senseless, unprovoked violence. Today's junk food is so devoid of the elements of life that what paltry bit of nutrition it does contain is only enough to fuel the limbic brain and not enough to fuel the higher brain. What do you want to bet that those two kids who shot up Columbine and then themselves were not on a diet rich in fruits and vegetables? I'll bet that everything they ever ate, especially outside of home, was some sort of junk or fast food.

Most of the things worth doing in the world had been declared impossible before they were done.

—Louis D. Brandeis

It must sound like I'm suggesting that kids should never again be allowed to eat Froot Loops or at McDonald's. I'm not. That would be unrealistic and ridiculous. You just can't tell kids that they can never have any of the foods they have been eating all their lives and are accustomed to having. But you can start to introduce living food and explain why. Some mornings give them a real fruit salad and tell them the difference between it and a bowl of Froot Loops, which likes to associate itself with fruit but is a totally worthless, disease-producing nonfood. Simply start. Do something. Let them know what you're doing and why, not with force, deprivation and inflexibility, but with love, understanding and patience. Sometime in the future they will thank you in a way they cannot even comprehend at present.

4. **I'm one of those who you describe as eating at best only 10 percent living food and 90 percent cooked food. Should I allow for some kind of transition period? Might I throw my body into turmoil if I change too radically too soon?**

One of the most interesting and impressive features of the living body is the fact that it is always, under any and all circumstances and conditions, striving to break down and remove toxins. Whether you are awake or asleep, in good health or poor, active or sedentary, the removal of wastes from the body is an activity that is ongoing to some degree twenty-four hours a day. We have already learned that the hours from 4:00 A.M. to 12:00 noon are when this activity is most heightened, but the removal of these toxins is so crucial to life that there is never a time when the body is not working, in some capacity at some level of effectiveness, to remove them. Your living habits, primarily what foods you eat, determine how much energy will be available for that continual effort. There is no question that when you alter your eating habits to eat more living food, which increases availability of energy, while simultaneously eating less cooked food, which decreases the expenditure of energy, toxins *will* start to be flushed from your body. Sometimes that can be uncomfortable and sometimes not, depending upon many variables that come into play, such as a person's genetic background, which determines overall strength and integrity of the body to perform all vital functions. This goes all the way back to how the person was fed in utero. A person's metabolism also plays a role: Is it weak or strong, effective or inefficient? Obviously, energy availability is a huge factor, as is the level of toxins that must be eliminated.

Over the years, I have seen it all. I have seen people who were on horrendous diets, eating practically *no* living food at all, who made a total and immediate turnaround to eating 70 percent or 80 percent living food and never experienced so much as a headache. They dropped weight; overcame, in some instances, catastrophic illness; eliminated pain; saw their energy skyrocket—all without the slightest discomfort. On the other side of the coin, I have seen people on bad diets, not horrible but in need of improvement, increase their intake of living food only moderately and have headaches and other bodyaches and feel so lethargic that they could hardly get around. They would flush toxins and lose weight, but they felt miserable. Not knowing all the variables interacting in your body, it would be impossible for me to state categorically if you will or will not experience discomfort if you make a quick and significant turnaround.

I can tell you that the vast majority of people, truly 75 to 80 percent, feel nothing negative; the other 20 to 25 percent do feel some kind of discomfort, everything from minor to major complaints. That's just the truth of the matter, and there's no sense in trying to pretend differently. Those who have a weak constitution and are highly toxic with lymph systems overburdened with wastes are likely to go through some initial discomfort that can last a week or even two. Any type of pain or ache, skin eruption, lethargy, diarrhea, irritability or other emotional upsets are possible. Doesn't sound like a great advertisement for living food, does it? But you must know that these symptoms are the result of the living body starting to cleanse and heal itself. Sometimes, with some people, that process is uncomfortable, and there's nothing that can be done about that. All I can tell you is that it will pass. At first, when the body has a newfound supply of energy to work with, it rushes headlong into the cleansing and elimination mode to get rid of as much waste as it can as quickly as possible, not knowing whether or not the newfound energy is a temporary phenomenon or if its availability will be ongoing. As soon as the body acclimates itself to having this energy on a regular basis, the discomfort subsides.

Patience and diligence, like faith, move mountains.

—WILLIAM PENN

The absolute worst possible thing you can do if you start to feel poorly is to go back to the way you were eating, which will only thwart your body's attempt to cleanse and heal itself. Once you commit and start, you must have faith in the wisdom of your body that it knows what it's doing and allow it to follow through on a process that *it has initiated* for its own well-being. This cleansing is absolutely essential before you can hope to lose weight permanently and feel renewed. The fact is, there are many people who are in dire need of a cleansing who make abrupt changes and not only experience no discomfort at all, but actually feel immense improvement in only four or five days.

I mentioned that you could have a bout with diarrhea, and I want to explain this further. Understand that over time a certain amount of waste will accumulate in the digestive tract. With the introduction of more living foods, which are around 90 percent water, the digestive tract is washed and flushed, resulting in diarrhea. Rarely does diarrhea last more than forty-eight hours, usually less. If the body is silted up with wastes and suddenly there's a lot of cleansing foods eaten, which living foods are, diarrhea is not at all surprising. Of course, if you experience diarrhea for longer than forty-eight hours, no matter what the cause or reason, you should check with your health-care practitioner immediately. But to experience it because you have introduced more cleansing, living food into your diet is not something to be alarmed about.

Remember, only a small percentage of people experience any uncomfortable symptoms. If you see them through, you will feel exhilarated and invigorated on the other side. It may be uncomfortable temporarily, but the feeling of renewal you will experience is well worth the effort.

5. **Now that I'm eating more fruits and vegetables, is it still necessary I drink eight glasses of water a day?**

Considering that water is the second most urgent need for life, second only to air, it is rather astonishing how few people fully recognize the devastating repercussions to the body when insufficiently hydrated, and the immeasurable good that results from properly meeting all of the body's water needs. I am aware that many people take too lightly the importance of drinking water, and there are even those whom I have heard say, "I don't drink water; it has no taste." Still, I was stunned to learn that according to one researcher, "75 percent of Americans are chronically dehydrated."[26]

It is impossible to overestimate the significance of

the role water plays in our lives. We are, after all, in the truest, most literal sense, water beings living on a water planet. From space our planet shines blue, distinguishing it from anything else in the universe. That blue color is the result of water. Some 70 percent of the planet Earth is water, and if it were not for the water, Earth would be a barren, lifeless rock, for water not only colors our planet, it also provides it with the capacity to harbor life. Remove water from a lush rainforest and you have a desert. Without water, no seed would germinate, no plant would grow, and no animal could live.

Without water, our bodies would be reduced to a few pounds of dust. For we, as is the planet, are about 70 percent water. The brain is more than 80 percent water; our blood, lymph fluid and saliva are more than 90 percent water. There is not a function of the body that does not depend on water. It is an essential part of every cell and all tissues and body fluids. Without water, you would have no saliva and could not swallow. Your tongue would stick to the inside of your mouth. Food would not be digested because digestive juices are practically all water. Every function of every organ depends on water. It holds nutrients in solution and transports them to the various parts of the body. It is water that picks up wastes and toxins from the cells via the lymph system and carries them to the organs of elimination. All of your inner organs swim in an ocean of fluids that is mostly water, without which, organs would stick together and tear. Water is the chief agent in regulating body temperature. It is the transport medium that carries everything we need into the body and to its cells and carries away all of the wastes we do not need.

Every day each of us loses about two quarts of water, at least. Depending on certain variables, it can easily be twice that amount. It is lost through perspiration and respiration. You lose water every time you exhale. Breathe on a window or a mirror and you can actually see the moisture from your lungs on the glass. You exhale many thousands of times every day, and each time you lose some water. This water *must be replaced every day,* and failing to do so will cause you more harm than you can possibly imagine. Depriving your body of its water needs, intentionally or unintentionally, negatively affects every activity and function of the living body, including that of losing weight.

So the question is, how much and what type? As far as how much water to drink, it is going to vary from person to person depending on certain variable conditions. Young or old, tall or short, male or female, physically active or sedentary, living in a hot or cold climate, and character of diet are all factors to consider. A significant amount of water is obtained through diet, so it stands to reason that if you increase the amount of living food you are eating, which contains mostly water, you will have less of a need than someone whose diet lacks living food.

For the sake of this discussion, when I say a glass, I'm talking about an eight-ounce glass. For as long as I can remember, the standard has been eight glasses of water a day. The reason is we lose approximately two quarts a day; a quart is thirty-two ounces, so eight 8-ounce glasses equals two quarts. But you have to take your own individuality into consideration when determining how much water you are going to drink. Obviously a person who lives in a hot climate or exercises vigorously or eats a lot of cooked food is going to require more water than someone who lives in a cold climate or is sedentary or eats mostly living food. You should take these differences into consideration. Eight glasses a day should be a generality, not an absolute.

In the same way you don't want to drink too little water, it is also not advisable to drink too much. Over-drinking water can waterlog tissues and dilute fluids. It also lowers the capacity of the blood to absorb and carry oxygen and impair cellular function. Do you know what happens to plants that are overwatered? It weakens them and can actually kill them. Nothing is gained by excessive water drinking, so use eight glasses a day as an average depending upon your own individual characteristics. On the whole, I'd say that since it's far more likely and easy to underdrink than overdrink, it would be better to have a little more than you need than not enough. The times when I would *always* have a glass of water are first thing in the morning upon awakening, right before eating a meal, and right before and right after exercising.

Considering that it's an established fact that at least two quarts of water are lost a day, not replacing that with a minimum of eight glasses of water a day is to risk your health and well-being. Another interesting aspect of this, which very few people realize, is that if you are trying to lose fat, water is essential to helping you do so. Even if you are doing absolutely everything right to lose weight and fat is released from your fat cells, if you do not drink enough water to flush that fat out of the body, the fat will remain in the bloodstream and eventually be stored back in your fat cells.

As far as what type of water to drink, my feeling is *anything* but tap water. I don't care who says what about how pure or how clean commercial "purified" tap water is, I wouldn't drink tap water unless there was absolutely no choice. Many people drink tap water without giving it a second thought. All manner of chemicals are added to water at purification plants, and that water picks up metallic contaminants merely by flowing through the intricate web of pipelines before reaching you. Almost all such water contains some chemical pollutants. DDT has been found in the far reaches of the North Pole. A host of chemicals, wastes, agricultural fertilizers and industrial pollutants all find their way into the water supply. To counteract this, other chemicals are deliberately added to the water supply to "purify" it and kill bacteria.

Today, the competition in the water market is intense. Like food, some water is pure, alive and wholesome, while some is lifeless, or worse—damaging. Aided by advanced water science and cutting-edge technology, a new class and generation of waters have been developed. These waters, with improved permeability and dissolvability, as well as enhanced nutritional value, have been designed to take us beyond merely surviving to actually thriving.

Our body's health is greatly affected by both the mineral and electrolyte balance of its fluids. (Electrolytes are responsible for the transfer of electrical energy in the body.) Therefore, if your water of choice has been cleansed, purified of all pollutants and undesirable natural and manmade contaminates—and then enhanced with a proper mineral and electrolyte formula—it becomes a superior vehicle for the replacement of minerals and electrolytes. Unlike most bottled and municipal tap water, which have a neutral pH, these waters are in an alkaline range, the same as human blood and other body fluids. This alkalinity not only helps maintain a proper acid–alkaline balance in the body, it also gives the water and extraordinarily velvety, silky smooth texture and a taste unlike any other.

For information on how to obtain this water or to learn more about the science of water, call toll free 1-877-215-1212, or visit *www.fitforlifetime.com* and click on Water.

6. **I have never been a big exercise buff. If I make the dietary changes you are suggesting and exercise only moderately, will I still see results?**

Absolutely! As long as you do some sort of exercise on a regular basis it will be enough to support your dietary changes. It will surprise you to learn how little exercise is actually needed. It is no exercise at all that makes it infinitely more difficult to see results. The relationship between a healthy life and regular exercise is irrefutable. And as far as losing weight is concerned, without some kind of regular exercise, you're just kidding yourself.

Those who think they have not time
for exercise will sooner or later
have to find time for illness.

—EDWARD STANLEY

It is best to do some exercise every day, if possible. If not, every other day is a must. Swimming, bicycling, jogging, rebounding or even a brisk walk will do the trick. My suggestion is a twenty- to thirty-minute walk each day. Walking is an ideal aerobic exercise to oxygenate the blood, which is crucial not only to weight loss, but to all health goals. Recent studies have shown that even the most moderate, unstructured walking programs will reap significant benefits.[27] Mile for mile, walking is actually the best fat burner. Walking four miles burns more fat than running the same distance in less time.[28] One scientific journal points out that a brisk, twenty-minute walk every other day produces substantial, recognizable benefits.[29] It also has been shown that the positive effects of walking are cumulative. So if you took three brisk ten-minute walks during the day, it would equal the results of one thirty-minute walk. Walking produces results in short-term training and in long-term health benefits equal to any other aerobic exercise, including jogging.[30]

Another good reducing exercise consists in placing both hands against the table edge and pushing back.

—ROBERT QUILLEN

It's hard to imagine that there is any health-conscious person anywhere who is not aware of the important role exercise plays in a healthy lifestyle. The benefits are enormous, everything from strengthening the heart[31] to increasing bone mass.[32] It lowers cholesterol,[33] helps with weight loss,[34] promotes better sleep,[35] reduces high blood pressure,[36] reduces back pain,[37] relieves stress,[38] and much more.

I want to tell you of another invaluable benefit of exercise that most people know nothing about. Earlier, in the chapter on the benefits that can be expected by eating more living food, I spoke of the far-reaching effect that the lymph system has on every area of a person's well-being and how important it is to the lymph system to be functioning at optimum efficiency. I also revealed that I felt my own life was saved from the effects of Agent Orange poisoning thanks to the efforts I made to cleanse my lymph system so that it could perform unhindered.

The cardiovascular system has at its center the heart, which is responsible for pumping the six quarts of blood through over 90,000 miles of blood vessels. Unlike the cardiovascular system, the lymph system has no such pump, even though it has to move three times more lymph than blood. Instead, it relies on physical activity—exercise. Movement, activity, physical exertion, that's what the lymph system depends upon to move lymph fluid through all the nodes, nodules, glands and vessels. And that is the number-one reason why exercise *must* be an integral part of your life if you wish to be successful at losing weight.

It would be a tragedy if you were to make the effort necessary to increase your intake of living food and decrease your intake of cooked food and then not also do whatever you could to assist and facilitate the mechanism specifically in charge of breaking down and removing excess weight from your body. From this point forward, whenever you hear the word "exercise" or even think of exercise, I would like for you to reflect on the inseparable link that exists between exercise, the lymph system and your quest to lose weight. Trying to lose weight without firing up your lymph system with exercise would be like trying to row your boat to shore without paddles.

7. **For some reason I can't seem to get it out of my head that I have to watch my calorie intake like a hawk or I'll never be successful at losing weight. Doesn't calorie counting help to some degree?**

Has it helped so far? Haven't those who are overweight been counting calories for decades in an attempt to lose weight? And hasn't it been unsuccessful? The problem of overweight is as bad as it's always been, if not worse. A fact of life is that myths die hard. It was once thought that tomatoes, being from the nightshade family, would kill you outright if you ate one. People wouldn't eat them because they didn't want to die to prove it. Finally, some brave fellow ate one "on the courthouse stairs" and survived. That myth was immediately put to rest. Other myths manage to hang on long past the time they should be retired.

Legend: a lie that has attained
the dignity of age.

—Laurence J. Peter

One dietary myth that held on with the obstinacy of a barnacle was the idea that if you didn't eat meat, the only way you could obtain all the necessary amino acids required to build protein was by some intricate, mazelike balancing act of eating different foods in just the right combination at each and every meal. No animal in nature has to combine different foods in a specific way in order to obtain the required amino acids and neither do we. The very idea that the Grand Planner would work things out so that unless we slaughtered and ate an animal we would have to go through a complicated, convoluted process of mixing and matching in order to obtain something as crucial to life as protein is patently asinine. Fortunately, that myth was disproved, recanted and thrown on the junk heap of history where it belongs. And the myth of "calories in and calories out" to lose weight needs to join it there. But there are still those who insist on clinging to these antiquated ideas. They remind me of those gray-suited Politburo guys who slammed their fists on the table saying, *"Nyet, nyet!"* to the idea of the USSR being broken up into different countries.

I am not the first person to ridicule the idea of calorie counting, nor is it a new subject of discussion. Consider the following by a more enlightened medical doctor in 1924: "The conception of the calorie has retarded logical and rational reasoning in regard to diet, more than any other single factor."[39]

One of the most outspoken and well-respected proponents of the calorie myth was the author of *The Rotation Diet*, Dr. Martin Katahn, director of the Weight Management Program at Vanderbilt University. In a follow-up book in 1989, *The T-Factor Diet,* he showed a lot of integrity by basically recanting his previous beliefs about the importance of the caloric value of foods and losing weight. He opened the book with, "A calorie is a calorie is a calorie, right? **WRONG!** New research in biochemistry shows that many of our old ideas about the caloric value of foods to the human body were wrong. All calories are not the same to the human body. When it comes to being overly fat or overweight, it's primarily the fat calories that count, *not* the carbohydrate and protein calories."[40]

Do you know what a calorie is? It's the amount of heat necessary to raise one gram of water one degree centigrade. A calorie is a measure of heat. It's not heat that makes you fat; it is, as Dr. Katahn says, *fat* that makes you fat.

One extremely relevant factor that is consistently left out of "a calorie is a calorie is a calorie" discussions is the nature of the food from which the calories are derived. A bowl of fruit can be high in calories, but because it's alive and has its enzymes intact, it requires no digestive effort from the body. Plus it's high in water, which helps flush toxins out. It there-fore has the effect of aiding weight loss when eaten correctly (alone on an empty stomach). A bowl of oatmeal can have fewer calories, but because it is cooked and lifeless it demands a greater effort from the body as it is forced to produce the enzymes it needs to digest. Plus it is practically devoid of water and is a heavy food that sits around for a long time as the body works on it.

Do yourself a favor: Let go of the calorie myth. It's a waste of time. You want to do some counting and figuring? Keep track of how much living food you eat and how much cooked food you eat. Don't allow the amount of cooked food to exceed living food, and you won't have to worry about being overweight for long.

Hey, have you ever noticed how thin people are

who live on or near the equator, the hottest part of our planet? If heat made you fat, wouldn't they be some of the heaviest people in the world instead of some of the thinnest? Just a thought.

8. **My doctor told me I have high blood pressure and suggested I go on Inderal. After looking over the side effects, I refused. Since I am overweight he suggested I lose weight to control it. Do you think this way of eating will help with my high blood pressure?**

I'd love to come right out and say, "Yes! By all means." But since I'm not a medical doctor, I have to be careful about statements like that. However, your doctor *did* tell you that you would be wise to lose weight, and that is something I can tell you this way of eating will achieve.

High blood pressure, or hypertension, occurs when the blood exerts too much pressure against the walls of the blood vessels. Fifty million people in the United States have high blood pressure, and it is the number-one risk factor for heart attacks and strokes.[41] It also causes brain damage and kidney failure, along with some other not-so-pleasant problems. Your doctor will tell you that in most people, the cause is unknown. However, some of the known risk factors are obesity, a diet high in saturated fat and salt, and a sedentary lifestyle. Your doctor will also tell you that he/she is stumped as to why even though there are a hundred drugs to control high blood pressure, only one-third of patients actually are able to keep it under control.[42] Obviously, drugs are not the answer.

I will tell you that over the years, literally hundreds of people have written letters to tell me that they have reduced their blood pressure into the normal range by eating according to my recommendations. Some have been able to discontinue their drugs and maintain normal blood pressure.

One such individual who had this kind of phenomenal success was a very close friend of mine who, coincidentally, was on Inderal for nearly ten years, yet his blood pressure was never in the normal range—it was only controlled so as not to kill him. After finally realizing that I was on to something with what I was studying, he started religiously following my approach to eating; his high blood pressure went to the normal range for the first time in ten years *without* the drugs. And it remained in the normal range.

For those of you with high blood pressure who are encouraged to read this and want to stop taking drugs, I wholeheartedly support you. However, it is exceedingly important that you don't abruptly stop taking the drugs even though you turn your diet completely around. There is a right way and a wrong way to get off drugs, and just suddenly stopping is the wrong way. The right way is to make the dietary changes you have learned here and have your physician monitor your success. As your blood pressure improves you can start to reduce your dosage of medication. By gradually going off the drugs you don't shock your system. In all likelihood, your physician would be happy for you to get your blood pressure in the normal range without drugs, and he/she will be able to decrease your dosage in the appropriate amounts until you are free of the drugs altogether.

9. **In the past I have taken appetite suppressants because no matter how much or how little I eat, I still feel hungry. I know the drugs are potentially harmful, so is there a natural appetite suppressant available?**

Yes, there is. I can tell you about the most natural appetite suppressant there is. It's called living food. Now, please don't think I'm being flippant or taking your concerns lightly. We all take delight from sitting down to a meal of delectable foods that look, smell and taste delicious, but let us never lose sight of the single most important reason why we eat. It is to supply the living body with what it needs to stay alive. All the rest of it—the enjoyment we reap from eating—is just a plus. The body requires nutrients and an energy source, and that is the biological and physiological reason why we eat. True hunger is the body's way of prompting us to take in the food, which ideally will have the nutrients and energy we need.

It stands to reason that the remarkably intelligent living body would have a mechanism in place to alert us that it is time to eat. How could it possibly be otherwise? After all, if we don't eat, we die. That mechanism is called the appestat, and it sits at the base of the brain like an alarm that goes on and off depending upon the level of need the body has. The appestat is constantly monitoring the bloodstream for nutrients and glucose. When it is determined that either or both are in short supply, the alarm is turned on, telling us to eat. When the bloodstream has a sufficient amount of nutrients and glucose, the alarm is shut off. (The only other time it shuts off is when the body is dealing with some health crisis, as related earlier.)

> A well-governed appetite is a
> great part of liberty.
>
> —SENECA

See if this doesn't sound familiar. Many people have told me that they frequently would eat a meal, then, even though they ate until satisfied, forty-five minutes later they were rooting around in the kitchen looking for something more to eat. They know they're not hungry; their stomachs are still full. Yet there they are, eating more food. I have even had people tell me that they *knew* they were overeating, but they couldn't help themselves. Something was making them seek out and eat more food. Can you relate?

There is actually a perfectly reasonable and under-standable explanation for this kind of counterproduc-tive behavior, and it has to do with the appestat. They ate meals so devitalized by cooking that the food did not contain enough nutrition to shut off the appestat. So even though their bellies were full, as far as the body was concerned, it needed food. Not that it actually needed food, but it did need nutrition, and food is the delivery system for bringing nutrition into the body. "Something" was telling them to eat. Living food is bursting with nutrition, both nutrients and carbohydrates, which are quickly converted to glucose, causing the appestat to shut off. That is why I said that living food is the most natural and healthy of appetite suppressants.

When people's diets are less than 10 percent living food and more than 90 percent cooked food, their appestats are clanging away at all hours of the day and night. The most tragic consequence of this is that it leads to overeating, and there is little else that is more destructive, more injurious or more of an impediment to losing weight than overeating. More than a hundred years ago, Sylvester Graham, an early practitioner of Natural Hygiene, said about overeating, "A drunkard may reach old age, a glutton never." More than 2,000 years ago, Hippocrates said, "Excess in drinking is *almost* as bad as excess in eating." Anyone who knows anything at all about health and how to acquire and maintain it will tell you that the most ruinous dietary habit of all is overeating. It overworks and poisons the body as it puts enormous stress and strain on all the organs, most especially the digestive system. And an impairment of digestion, which overeating inevitably causes, leads not only to overweight, but also to the overall breakdown of the body. Even the most wholesome food is spoiled when overeaten. Overeating also stretches the stomach so much that when it empties, you feel like there's a cavern that needs filling. Fortunately the stomach shrinks when meals are more reasonably sized. Eat until you're full, then stop.

I saw few die of hunger; of eating,
a hundred thousand.

—BENJAMIN FRANKLIN

We are unfortunately trained and conditioned to overeat at an early age. I know it's well-meaning, but telling a child who has had enough food and instinctively stops eating to "clean your plate if you want dessert" is the worst possible message that can ever be given. It forces children to overeat and accustoms them to the habit. Those are the children who wind up in Overeaters Anonymous when they are grown. Overeating is the greatest culprit of all in undermining health. Don't do it! Living food will help break the habit.

When it comes to eating,
you can sometimes help yourself
more by helping yourself less.

—RICHARD ARMOUR

I know there are other factors involved in over-eating. Our emotions get all tangled up with eating, and we wind up eating for all the wrong reasons. If you can find out what emotional and psychological factors are at work in causing you to overeat, you will be doing yourself a great service. Do whatever you have to do to stop overloading your stomach. You would be far better off having four or five small meals during the day than two or three larger meals that are overeaten.

What you will come to realize is that the longer you accustom your body to living food, the easier it becomes to normalize your eating habits and bring them in line with your goals of weight loss and improved health. Think about it: What greater ally could you hope to have than the intelligence that governs not only the activities of your body but all of life? Living food unleashes this intelligence so that it can go to work on your behalf. Living food helps the living body live well.

10. **I am hypoglycemic, and I'm wondering how this way of eating impacts on that condition.**

Another way of describing hypoglycemia is low blood sugar. Do you recall the importance that was put on having sufficient glucose in the bloodstream in the chapter on fruit? Glucose is the primary fuel for all body tissues. Because brain energy stores are very small, a constant supply of glucose must always be available to maintain adequate brain function. It is, therefore, imperative that the blood glucose level be maintained. If it's not, and insufficient glucose is available, a person will experience irritability, fatigue, nervousness, headache and general discomfort.

Those with low blood sugar are advised by their physicians to carry with them at all times some type of candy or sugar packets to be consumed when needed. That's the Band-Aid mentality: It does nothing to address the underlying problem. If one of the tires on your car kept going flat, which do you think would be the best course of action? To carry a pump with you and fill the tire every time it emptied, then drive on it until it needed to be filled again? Or seal the leak?

I have told you throughout this book that when it comes to diet and the living body, there are generally certain variables and contributing factors that come into play with different individuals. That is why it is difficult in the extreme to make sweeping, blanket statements. However, it has been my experience that those people with the garden variety of hypoglycemia, in other words *not* those dealing with some kind of diabetic situation or impaired pancreatic function, can rather easily avoid low blood sugar. You see, it's mighty hard to have low blood sugar if there's sufficient sugar in the blood. Fructose, the sugar component in fruit, is transformed to glucose immediately, with less effort required from the body than for anything else you might eat. By eating fruit in the manner described, which means fresh, alone and on an empty stomach, the bloodstream will have a nice steady supply of glucose.

Frequently, people have told me that all they have

to do to end a hypoglycemic attack is eat some protein. Let me explain why this works. A hypoglycemic attack is the body reacting to being deprived of the glucose-producing carbohydrates it requires. That reaction requires energy. When a heavy food such as protein enters the stomach, energy is diverted there to deal with it, *temporarily* relieving the symptoms of hypoglycemia. But as soon as the initial stages of digestion are completed, the body gets back to what it was doing, which was alerting you to the glucose shortage. The symptoms return. Eating protein every two to three hours does nothing to end hypoglycemia; it only forestalls it. By making fruit a regular part of your diet and utilizing the three Keys to Success, you remove the *cause* of hypoglycemia rather than constantly battling its symptoms.

CHAPTER ELEVEN

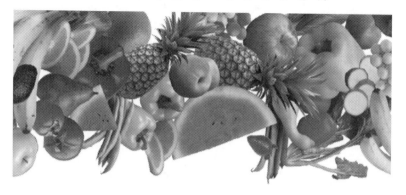

FORM A PARTNERSHIP

Nothing can withstand the
onslaught of laughter.

—MARK TWAIN

A few years ago the pope was invited, on very short notice, to attend a world conference on peace at the United Nations in New York. He graciously accepted and was told it would not start until he arrived as his presence would lend such credibility to the gathering.

The pope landed at the airport in New York and was picked up by a driver in a magnificent limousine, as befitting his stature. As the driver helped the pope into the back seat, he asked if there was anything he could do to make him more comfortable. The pope answered, "Thank you, my son, this is more than fine, but I am due at the United Nations and I'm a bit late, so if you could possibly expedite this trip, I would appreciate it immensely."

"Just sit back and relax, Your Holiness," said the driver, "I know this city well, and I'll have you there in no time."

Off they went, and in less than ten minutes they were stuck in the middle of some of New York's famous traffic, unable to move.

"Excuse me, my son," said the pope. "Ordinarily, I wouldn't say anything, but I must be at the United Nations. Many people are waiting for me."

"I'm so sorry, Your Grace," answered the driver, "but there's little I can do."

"Would you mind if I tried?" asked the pope.

"Try what, Your Grace? You mean, can you drive?"

"Yes, I would like to drive."

The driver was bewildered, but said, "Of course, anything you wish, Your Holiness."

So they switched places, and the pope got in the driver's seat, shifted the gear into low and, with two tires up on the sidewalk he traveled past the cars that were stopped. He burst through the gate of a closed parking lot, came out on the other side and headed down a one-way street in the wrong direction. He was now making good time. Right about then, one of New York's Finest pulled the limousine over. The officer got out of his car and, rather agitated at the liberties someone was taking in a big, beautiful limousine, walked up to the driver's window only to see the pope sitting there in full regalia.

"Your Holiness!" said the officer.

"Please, my son, I'm needed at the United Nations. Can you please help me?"

The officer was dumbstruck but managed to say, "Yes, of course, Your Holiness, but I must call my chief first, then I'll give you a police escort all the way. I'll be right back."

"Thank you, my son."

The officer dashed to his squad car, called in, and the following conversation ensued between the officer and his chief:

"Chief, you will not guess in a thousand years who I just pulled over."

"Who is it? What did you do, stop the mayor?"

"No, no, Chief, you're not thinking big. Think *big*."

"Don't play games with me. Just tell me who it is. What did you do, stop the governor?"

"No, Chief, you're still not thinking big enough. This is *huge!*"

"Look, I don't have time for this. Just tell me, is it the president of the United States?"

"No, Chief, you're still not getting it. Think the *biggest* of the big."

"Hey, cut the games, and tell me who it is right now, or you'll find yourself walking a beat."

"I don't know who it is, Chief, but his chauffeur is the *pope!*"

Can you guess the message of this little tale? Things aren't always what they appear to be on the surface. And that, I can tell you, is the case when it comes to successfully losing weight and keeping it off. For those who have tried and tried and tried again to lose weight and were either unsuccessful or managed to slim down only to put it all back on again, it most certainly does appear on the surface that it's a hopeless struggle. And when statistics show that 90 percent of dieters put the weight back on that they managed to lose, and that the problem of overweight continues to worsen year after year, it's no wonder so many people can't lose weight and think it's an ongoing battle that can't be won.

The deepest personal defeat suffered
by human beings is constituted by the
difference between what one was
capable of becoming and what
one has in fact become.

—ASHLEY MONTAGU

But aren't some people successful? Aren't there those who manage to figure out the right combination of factors that allow them to enjoy long-term success? *I'm* one. I've managed to learn how to keep my weight in check even though I'm a hardcore food junkie who loves to eat, and I'm not unique or special in any way. If anything, the ease with which I put on weight could easily have put me into the category of the permanently rotund. Don't you know some people who have managed to figure it out? Aren't there celebrities or other people in the public eye who you've seen lose weight and keep it off? The point I'm trying to make is that it *can* be done. It's just a matter of hitting the right combination of factors that ultimately results in success.

The most obvious area of need is on the physical plane. It is our physical bodies that we want to have control over and keep in good shape. I don't want to imply that I have *the* answer, or the best answer or the only answer. But I have figured out *an* answer. It's one that honors life and provides the body with all the constituents of health that are the prerequisites of life. Everything that the living body needs to stay alive and flourish is in living food—every last vitamin, of which there are many; every last mineral, of which there are also many; the full complement of amino acids to build protein; the most easily utilizable carbohydrates and sugars for energy; all the intact digestive enzymes so the body doesn't have to manufacture its own; all the phytonutrients, antioxidants and other compounds and substances that promote life and are required by the living body—all are naturally occurring in living food.

Living food is also pleasing to all the senses, has a high water content, is slightly alkaline rather than acid and is environmentally friendly.

I have endeavored throughout the course of this book to show you how to integrate living food into your eating lifestyle in an easygoing way that will not *only* help you lose weight, but also allow you to enjoy the eating experience, to eat the foods you like, to avoid crash diets, and to refrain from resorting to drugs, absurd devices that fly in the face of reason or powdered drinks instead of food. All of this, plus it nurtures, supports and improves your overall health and well-being. I've watched this approach work for hundreds of thousands of people over the last thirty-plus years, and there is not the slightest doubt in my mind that you can join their ranks if you will apply what you have learned and give it a fair trial.

It has often been stated that the most prominent difference between human beings and other animal beings is our ability to think. We can take in huge amounts of data, differentiate it, categorize it, apply what we have learned or experienced in the past, and determine in the present what we will do in the future. This is nonexistent in other animal beings, making us unique. We can think! And thinking plays an immense, incalculable role in our lives.

Change your thoughts and you
change your world.

—Norman Vincent Peale

What would you say is the message of the following statements? You are what you think you are; it is done unto you as you believe; when you think it, you will be it; all that you are is the result of what you have thought; when you believe it, you will see it; if you can think it, you can be it; as you think, so shall you be. I could go on as there are numerous more examples. I'm pretty sure that the message is that there is a lot more to life than the physical world we relate to with the physical senses. The physical world is but a part of life. We also exist in a mental world—a world that we don't relate to with sight, sound, smell, taste or touch but is every bit as real as the physical world. The mental world's center is everywhere; its circumference is nowhere.

Is there any doubt in your mind that gravity is real? Any at all? You certainly cannot see, hear, smell, taste or touch gravity. But you know it exists, don't you? If not, all you would have to do is hold an anvil over your bare foot and let go. You would then have an obvious and undeniable, albeit painful, illustration of the law of gravity in action. Well, there are laws in the mental/thinking world that are just as unyielding as the law of gravity.

Every good thought you think
is contributing its share to the ultimate
result of your life.

—GRENVILLE KLEISER

Our mental attitude plays a big role in our lives on every level, and that's what I'd like to address here. A good example of what I'm talking about can be illustrated with sports figures. There's no doubt that Tiger Woods can hit a golf ball 300 yards right down the center of the fairway. There's no doubt that Barry Bonds can hit a baseball out of the ballpark. Michael Jordan can swish a basketball through the hoop from twenty feet. Andre Agassi can hit a tennis ball where his opponent isn't. Bret Favre can throw touchdown passes, and Wayne Gretzky can score goals. But do they do it every time? No. Why not? They absolutely have the physical ability and attributes to do it every time, but they don't. Why? I have heard every one of the sports stars mentioned above, and numerous others as well, attribute their success or failure not to their physical prowess, but to their mental attitude. Over and over again before and after competitions, I have heard athletes make comments like, "If my mental game is there, I'll be fine," or "I was mentally strong today, and that's why I came out on top." I have *rarely* ever heard an athlete praise his or her physical strength. It is almost always about their mental state. It is my belief that anything we do in the physical world can be affected by our mental attitude, whether it's hitting a ball or losing weight.

When I spoke about the law of gravity and said there are also laws in the mental/thinking world, I was referring specifically to the Law of Attraction. When you hear someone say, "Like attracts like," or "Birds of a feather flock together," the person is referring to the Law of Attraction. Probably the most well-known and recognizable comment is, "You reap what you sow." At the time those words were spoken, you couldn't just amble over to the corner grocery store if you were hungry. If you didn't grow food, you didn't eat, so reaping and sowing was a most well-understood term that no one could possibly misconstrue. In other words, if you want grapes, you had better plant grape seeds. Plant thistles, and there will be no grapes, only thistles, which are a lot harder to chew and swallow than grapes, and are not nearly as tasty. Obviously, those who lived on the land and depended upon agriculture for their survival knew that they could only harvest what they planted. The statement was spoken as a parable. In other words, it was meant to be a teaching tool for all aspects of life.

It is the height of absurdity to sow little but weeds in the first half of one's lifetime and expect to harvest a valuable crop in the second half.

—PERCY JOHNSTON

The Law of Attraction, as described by "you reap what you sow," also exists and is as real in the mental/thinking world as it is in the physical world. Thoughts become things as surely as seeds become plants. That is why beautiful Jesus said over and over in so many different ways, "It is done unto you as you believe." He wasn't a practical jokester or a prankster trying to leave messages to mislead or trick people. No, I think that whether Jesus plays a big role in your life or none at all, most people would agree that he had a desire to assist people and help them live a more fulfilling life. Thus, his most recognizable statement about turning your beliefs into reality was designed to help people obtain that which they truly desire.

So what do you believe about yourself? How do you describe your condition? Do you ever refer to yourself in a negative or unflattering way? Do your thoughts and comments about yourself empower and support you, or weaken and discourage you?

Have you ever heard someone say, out of frustration or disappointment, things like, "It's hopeless; I'll never be able to lose weight," or "I've always been fat, and I'll always be fat," or "It's no use, no matter what I try doesn't work," or "I guess it's just in the stars for me to fail," or "It doesn't matter what I do or how hard I try, I'm just destined to be overweight," or any number of other defeatist statements? If the Law of Attraction is real, if what you believe truly is done unto you, if you do indeed reap what you sow, do you think statements like that in any way, shape or form further your efforts and help achieve the desired goal? Think of the people you respect and admire for what success they've had and achievements they've made in any area of life. Do you think they fill their heads with negative, defeatist comments or positive, supportive ones?

In the beginning of this book, I spoke about the infinite intelligence that governs all of life. The intelligence that keeps the planet Earth on its correct axis. The intelligence that gave us life and directs every activity, large or small. The intelligence that gave birds flight and the rose its scent.

This intelligence is everywhere. It operates in, around and through us, and *it is on your side*. The universe isn't working against you; it's working *for* you.

You are a physical being and a mental being. The physical and mental parts of your life are like the two sides of a coin. They are inseparably intertwined. What you do to or for one, you do to the other. A person who doesn't feel well physically, either because of excess weight or any other physical challenge, is likely to also have a negative mental attitude, and it's a downward spiral. But that spiral can just as easily be reversed. Any road traveled in one direction can be traveled in the opposite.

I am the master of my fate; I am
the captain of my soul.
　　　　　　　　　　—W. E. HENLEY

I have set forth within these pages an effective, common-sense, easily doable approach to help you lose weight and feel better physically. It's up to you to complete the circle. Along with changing your diet in terms of the way you eat, in order to be truly successful, you must also change your mental diet in terms of the way you think. Instead of all those negative, disempowering statements, what if you fed your mind affirmative, uplifting messages? You are the master of your thoughts. You can choose to think anything you want to think. One of the most glorious aspects of being a human being is that you have freedom of choice. You can react to any situation in any way you please. Your well-being isn't determined by what happens to you in life. It's determined by the way you *react* to what happens to you in life. *You* are in control. *You* are in charge, and when you start to feed those type of positive messages into your consciousness on a regular basis, good things start to happen.

You can align yourself with the intelligence of the universe. What do you think is the tool of intelligence? *Thought*. Your thoughts can put you in harmony with this intelligence and have it work for you. You're already thinking something. Since you have a choice, what if you were to make statements like this: "I am the child of a loving God who *wants* me to be happy and fulfilled"; "Everything I need to be successful in my life is available to me"; "Losing weight and getting my health in order aren't only for other people; they're for me, too"; "I can do whatever I set my mind to do"; "I am a good person, and I am worthy of good in my life"; "There are people in my life whom I love and who love me"; "Circumstances don't rule my life; I do." I'm not talking about wishful thinking here, or saying these things by rote in the hope that it will make a difference. I'm talking about replacing fear, worry and doubt in your life with faith, trust and belief.

Remember, happiness doesn't
depend on who you are or what you have;
it depends solely on what you think.

—DALE CARNEGIE

Living food is right for your body, and affirmative thoughts are right for your mind. It's a winning combination that can't be beat. As you start to lose weight and see progress in that area, you will naturally feel good about yourself and be more inclined to complement that success with uplifting, supportive thoughts. The body helps the mind; the mind helps the body. Upwards you go until you realize all of your goals. A healthy body and mind fling open the door to success and happiness, and *you* are the possessor of the key that unlocks that door.

I wrote this book to help you—to lose weight, yes, but also to bring about a significant improvement in your overall health. Obviously, it is my wish that you will resonate with the information it contains, take it to heart and implement the changes it suggests. If you do, I know you will reap the rewards. In either event, wherever you go and whatever you do, may God bless your every breath and guide your every step.

APPENDIX I:
MINERALS FOR LIFE

If anything is sacred,
the body is sacred.

—Walt Whitman

Your body is able to manufacture some vitamins, but it cannot make any of the minerals that are necessary for life. You must obtain an abundant supply of food-grade minerals from your diet, and if you don't, all manner of health problems can result, both minor and major. Since most people I've known know precious little about minerals, I'm going to lay out a few interesting and pertinent facts about them. First of all, we still do not know all the minerals that are present and utilized within the body. There are between twenty-five and thirty that have definite and known uses and about a dozen more whose uses are not fully understood. There are some found in appreciable quantities within the body, including calcium, magnesium, phosphorous and iron. Most minerals are called "trace minerals" because of the minute amount present in the body, such as zinc, cobalt, silver and boron.

There is definitely confusion as to what type of minerals can and cannot be used by the body. Most knowledgeable people recognize that the body must have certain minerals to accomplish its work and preserve health. However, only a few realize that these minerals must be in their organic state to do us any good.

Here are the facts: (1) Minerals are inorganic as they exist naturally in the soil and water; (2) minerals are organic as they exist in plants and animals; (3) only plants or animals can transform inorganic minerals into organic minerals; (4) animals are poor converters of inorganic minerals because they are engineered to get their minerals from plants or by eating other animals; (5) inorganic minerals are only poorly absorbed (about 5 percent) and can be injurious to animals.

Because inorganic and organic minerals have the same *chemical* composition, they were confused by early researchers. They mistakenly assumed that a chemical similarity in minerals also meant there was a nutritive similarity. Big mistake. It's true that, chemically, iron in the bloodstream and iron in nails are the same, and that calcium in rocks (dolomite) is identical to calcium in the bones. But it is a grave error to believe that the body can digest, assimilate and utilize powdered nails and crushed rocks.

The number-one mineral, *by quantity*, needed by the human body is calcium. Calcium is biochemically necessary to life, crucial to health and instrumental in keeping you flexible and youthful.

Over time, the average person becomes more and more depleted of calcium. By age forty, over 50 percent of Americans are severely calcium-deficient; by age sixty, over 90 percent are calcium-deficient. These drastic declines show that the majority of Americans are not obtaining enough *utilizable* calcium from their diets. What I mean by utilizable is that it is in a form that can be absorbed and assimilated by the body. For that to occur the calcium must be "ionized," or it is worthless.

When minerals enter your body they interact with certain stomach secretions that render them capable of being absorbed. This process is called ionization. Every mineral you ingest must undergo ionization in your stomach before it can be assimilated. The body *must* reduce any form of dietary or supplemental calcium into calcium ions. These ion-charged particles of calcium are the *only* form of calcium the body is able to metabolize, and thereby absorb and have available for use.

If you don't obtain enough ionized calcium in your diet, especially from fruits and vegetables, the body will leach calcium from the bones, the only place it can, so it can neutralize acid. This leads directly to the dreaded osteoporosis.

The organic calcium in fruits and vegetables is already ionized, but most people don't eat nearly the amount of fruits and vegetables they should, so they resort to dairy products and/or calcium supplements. What could possibly be more obvious than the fact that dairy products and supplements simply are not the answer? Although Americans are one of the biggest dairy-eating populations in the world, they also continue to have one of the highest incidences of osteoporosis. Although the calcium in cow's milk is ionized from the cow, once it's subjected to the blistering heat of pasteurization the calcium is deranged and very little of it can be absorbed. Pasteurization kills and destroys everything of worth.

As far as taking calcium supplements, they are typically poorly ionized. For example, calcium citrate, made from crushed rocks, is only about 15 percent ionized. Calcium gluconate, also made from crushed rocks, is worse, only about 5 percent ionized. *We are not rock eaters.*

I would call milk perhaps the most unhealthful vehicle for calcium that one could possibly imagine.

—NEAL BARNARD, M.D.

Trying to obtain the calcium your body needs from dairy products and supplements can have some very detrimental repercussions. Unfortunately, over the years, the mind-set has been that taking in extra calcium from dairy or supplements is a harmless precaution. It isn't! In fact, it's disease-producing. Trying to fulfill the body's requirements for calcium with nonionized calcium *will not work*. If your car requires premium, high-octane fuel and you fill the tank with diesel fuel, what do you think will happen? True, they're both fuels, but only one can be used by your car. It's not a harmless mistake. The car won't run, and the diesel will damage the engine.

The extra calcium that is not used by the body isn't harmlessly eliminated. It is picked up by the blood and deposited in the soft tissue—the blood vessels, skin, eyes, joints and internal organs. Unused calcium combines with fat and cholesterol in the blood vessels to cause hardening of the arteries. The calcium that ends up in the skin causes wrinkling. In the joints, it crystallizes and forms painful arthritic deposits. In the eyes, it takes the form of cataracts, and in the kidneys it forms kidney stones. Hardly a harmless practice. Are these maladies that I just listed not prevalent in the United States? Are they not right on par with our overconsumption of nonutilizable calcium?

There is another extremely important consideration that has to be taken into account, which over the years has been routinely misunderstood and overlooked. A mineral deficiency rarely exists in a vacuum. The study of minerals by themselves necessarily leads to a fragmented view of nutrition. Minerals have an interdependence with many other various elements of food and with the complex actions of the body itself. Minerals are *not* isolated food factors but rather parts of the nutritional whole. No mineral is used in isolation within the body. All minerals interact with other minerals.

This is so elemental as to stun the intellect; so few people grasp this simple but obvious fact of life. The way it has been set up by the intelligence that has been noted and praised throughout this book is that minerals are created in concert with other cofactors in food and are intended to be ingested in that way. Still, owing in large part to the error of confusing organic, ionized minerals with inorganic, non-ionized ones because they are chemically the same, the habit of ingesting isolated, fragmented calcium persists.

If you've ever made rice, you know that the amount of water and amount of rice has a certain correct ratio. It is, in fact, a ratio of 2:1, or two cups of water for each cup of rice. If that 2:1 ratio is not adhered to, the rice will not come out properly. Too much or too little of either the water or the rice and you will wind up with rice that is either mushy and sticky or burnt and dry.

Would it interest you to know that in order for calcium to be effectively absorbed and utilized in the body, it has to not only be ionized but also must be in the presence of magnesium? It also requires certain trace minerals, but magnesium is the primary cofactor that calcium needs to be useable by the body. And the ratio of calcium to magnesium is the same as water to rice, or 2:1.

I can assure you that neither dairy products nor the vast majority of commercial supplements have calcium that is ionized or in the proper ratio of 2:1 calcium to magnesium. Even if certain calcium supplements have the correct amount of magnesium added, it is unlikely to be ionized. So on and on it goes, with Americans loading up on more than 125 billion pounds of dairy products a year and hundreds of millions of dollars worth of calcium supplements, and still problems associated with a calcium deficiency, most notably osteoporosis, are rampant. Is it working? No, it is not working, and proof that it is not is sadly right before our eyes.

I'm not writing this section for the sole purpose of loading you up with a bunch of bad news. Nor do I wish to leave you feeling hopeless that you can't help support the calcium needs of your body with a high-quality, nontoxic supplement that fully meets all the specific requirements necessary to be effective. On the contrary, I want to tell you about an amazing discovery that will surely revolutionize the entire calcium-supplement industry.

In 1979, a British journalist went to Japan to interview one of the oldest documented living people in the world, Mr. Izumi. He was a sprightly 115-year-old man in amazingly good health who lived on an island off the coast of Japan. He was healthy, active and alert. Many of the other inhabitants on the island were also in great health and seldom died before age ninety-five.

Researchers found the water the islanders drank was uniquely different. It contained ionized minerals leached from living coral on which the island was built. These unique coral minerals made the water highly alkaline. When drunk it helped the body keep a superior acid–alkaline balance. If you will recall, earlier in the book I pointed out that the human bloodstream is slightly alkaline and must stay in the alkaline range. However, the American diet is highly acidic, so there is a constant need for the body to neutralize this acid, and calcium is leached from the bones to do so.

Because the living coral ingests a large spectrum of natural, sun-radiated minerals from the ocean water, powder made from the coral contains a rich concentration of these naturally occurring minerals. Here's the truly exciting part of this discovery: These coral minerals are the only source in the world of minerals that are naturally in a highly ionized state (up to 92 percent!). Plus, the coral's large amounts of both ionized calcium and magnesium naturally occur in the *exact right ratio of 2:1*. And if that were not enough, it also contains the necessary trace minerals such as zinc, copper and manganese, also in ionized form, and is free of toxic metals such as lead, mercury, cadmium and arsenic.

This favored species of coral also contains a harmless form of aluminum; this form of aluminum occurs naturally in the same form found in literally all fruits and vegetables (not the dangerous form found in toxic dental restorative materials and associated with memory problems).

I started to notice that these "coral calciums" were being aggressively marketed in magazines, infomercials and through multilevel marketing. Like everything else that is marketed to the public, I know that there are inferior and superior products of all kinds. I wanted to know which one of the coral calciums was the absolute, unrivaled best of the best, so I did precisely what I did when I wanted to locate the finest and purest Live Plant Enzymes: I conferred with the most knowledgeable and well-respected authorities in the world of nutritional research, those people to whom the experts go for dependable, definitive answers.

Did you know that research shows that you have only a 2.5 percent chance of selecting a nutritional product in the marketplace that is both nontoxic and effective? In other words, you have a 97.5 percent chance of selecting a nutritional product that is either toxic or doesn't work.

This rather shocking statistic was confirmed in a landmark study reported in the *Journal of the American Nutraceutical Association* (Winter 1999).

If you are taking, or want to take, a coral calcium, you should take several critical factors into consideration, and ask about them from whomever you are obtaining the product.

First, you should know that not all corals are equal. Not by a long shot. There are 2,500 different species of coral worldwide with varying mineral contents and levels of ionization. Some contain calcium and almost no magnesium at all. Surprisingly, only *one* form contains naturally occurring magnesium in the ideal 2:1 calcium to magnesium ratio. Make sure you check the ingredients, and here's what to look for: Let's say, for example, in the ingredients listed it shows "calcium from coral—400 mg." That means since there is 400 mg of calcium there has to be 200 mg of magnesium. If it lists "magnesium from coral—200 mg" it is from the correct species. But if it shows, "magnesium from coral plus some other magnesium source, such as magnesium carbonate—200 mg," it's not the best coral. The magnesium carbonate had to be added to bring the magnesium level up to the correct balance. The carbonate will not be ionized, so this would be an inferior product.

Also, you want to check to see if there are any flowing agents added such as silicone dioxide, which is sand, or magnesium stearate, which is toxic hydrogenated oil and creates trans fats known to cause elevated cholesterol levels. Death from heart disease and cancer have been reported to be highest among consumers of this type of fat.

You should also find out if the powder is ground by nickel-free grinders to retain the value of the coral and avoid any toxic nickel residues.

Find out also if isolated trace minerals have been added that have poor bioavailability. In the correct species of coral these are naturally occurring and highly bioavailable.

Last, vitamin D_3 is essential for proper calcium absorption and it occurs naturally in the correct species of coral. If you see "vitamin D_3 as cholecalciferol," you know it is synthetic.

The marine coral I researched meets all of these criteria, making it the finest coral-calcium product on the market today.

Ordinarily I would not encourage anyone to take a calcium supplement because I know that living food can supply our calcium needs and most calcium supplements simply do not make the grade. Since coral was once living, it thereby can transform minerals into an organic, highly ionized state. The fact is that the product I researched uses exclusively the species of coral that has the correct 2:1 calcium-to-magnesium ratio, and it is harvested and formulated under the strictest, most pristine conditions that result in a most superior product. For this reason I will tell you that if you wish to take a calcium supplement that is the purest, safest, highest-quality product available, this is the one you can have complete and total confidence in. You can find out how to obtain the coral calcium I have described here by calling toll free 1-877-942-4492 or 1-877-215-1212. For more information:

Web site: *www.fitforlifetime.com*
e-mail: *info@fitforlifetime.com*

APPENDIX II:
WHAT HAS HAPPENED
TO COMMON SENSE?

There's many a mistake
made on purpose.

—THOMAS HALIBURTON

It is with great sadness and bitter disappointment that I write this section of the book. But I have no choice in the matter because, unfortunately, circumstances demand that I do so. There is an insidious scam afoot that threatens to severely undermine your health and the health of everyone you know and love. It is something so excruciatingly outrageous that it's hard to imagine any sane person not becoming enraged and infuriated upon learning of the scheme. But as is often the case when it comes to money, even those who are sane will endorse the insane when the price is right. And the people responsible for this diabolical assault against your well-being have all the money they need to hire the most highly credentialed apologists and spin-doctors on the market—those people who would violate any trust, attempt any subterfuge, concoct any sham, fabricate any lie, pervert any truth and disseminate any misinformation in order to plump up their bank accounts.

And all the while they feign indignation at having their integrity questioned as they flap their sacred credentials in your face, as though that is all they require to have their word taken as gospel no matter how disingenuous their true motives may be.

The only place any rationally thinking person would expect to hear of what I am referring to is from a deranged lunatic or from some unthinkable Hollywood science-fiction or horror movie. But this is not fiction; it is all too true, I'm afraid. And it is riddled with lies, deception, conniving, duplicity and, of course, gigantic corporate profits. So, what do you think? Can you tell it's something I'm not particularly enamored with, or have I not let my true feelings be known? The reason I am taking such an aggressive stance and using such strong language is that this is not something to be taken lightly. It is not a time to tiptoe around the issue using phony niceties so as not to offend anyone.

This book has been written to help you attain a higher level of well-being by shedding excess weight while simultaneously improving your overall health. Your success depends on *one* guiding principle, *one* course of action that will help you prevail in your quest and accomplish your goal. It is simply this: Supply your living body with more living food than dead food. That's it. Dead food is, of course, food that has been cooked or otherwise processed so as to destroy the life force (enzymes) in the food. It is my contention that the primary reason obesity and overweight are at such epidemic levels—why cardiovascular disease and cancer are the two top killers in our country, taking one and a half million lives every year—is that Americans eat far more cooked food than living food. It is a trend that *must* be reversed in order to reverse the dire statistics. Every effort should be made to educate people and help them see the need to increase the amount of living food and decrease the amount of cooked (dead) food in their diet.

Perhaps you can fully appreciate and be able to understand my outrage and incendiary language when I tell you what has been going on. The power brokers willing to sacrifice your health on the altar of profits have used their considerable wealth and influence to devise a scheme whereby they make lots of money and you are *unable* to purchase any living food whatsoever. Not a bite. You will only be able to obtain dead food unless it is organically grown or you grow it in your own backyard. Everything else will be rendered dead before you buy it. Unless you have already figured out what I am talking about, you must be thinking, *That's crazy! First of all, who in their right mind would even want to kill all living food, and second of all, the American people would never stand for such lunacy.* That's what you think. **It's already happening!**

And just wait until you hear what the food is being treated with to kill it. You had better brace yourself. **NUCLEAR WASTE!** Yes, I'm serious—*dead* serious, and no, you are not in the middle of a nightmare from which you are about to awaken. This is all too real. Let me ask you

a question. What was your immediate, instantaneous reaction to reading that all the food you and your family will
ever eat is going to first be treated with nuclear waste?
Were you joyous at the prospect, or were you repulsed? Did
it seem like a perfectly natural thing to do, or something
you wouldn't even joke about doing? Did it resonate with
your common sense, or did you instinctively recoil at the
idea? Because you are going to have to rely on your sense of
logic, reason, common sense and instincts on this one. The
proponents of food irradiation, and that is what I am talking about here, are hoping you won't. They are hoping you
will believe the lies and propaganda they are expertly dis-
seminating to lull you into complacency so you will accept
this horror of the Nuclear Age and go along with it like so
many sheep.

In propaganda, as in advertising,
the important consideration is not whether
information accurately describes an
objective situation, but whether
it sounds true.

—CHRISTOPHER LASCH

No matter what you have already heard about food irradiation, and no matter what you may hear about it in the
future, don't ever lose sight of the fact that it is nuclear
waste that would be used on your food. Those who want to
avoid that fact will attempt to couch it in seemingly benign

terms in order to throw you off. They will prop up "world-renowned experts" to allay your fears and try to discredit people who are willing to speak out against it. They will describe it in vague terms, using quaint euphemisms that are less objectionable than the truth, but no amount of camouflage and whitewashing will alter the fact that it is *nuclear waste* they are trying to make less objectionable. You can call rat meat filet mignon, but that doesn't make it so.

Remember earlier in the book when I cited the two impeccably conducted studies that appeared in the same issue of the *New England Journal of Medicine* that came to exactly *opposite* conclusions? This section I'm writing could easily dissolve into a long, drawn-out and boring battle of "my studies versus your studies." Frankly, it would be a waste of time. Instead of relying on studies about what may or may not be known, I'm going to stick to that which is already verifiably known. Hopefully, after you have had a chance to contemplate the facts, rather than the factitious, your common sense will rule your thinking on the matter.

Surely one of your first questions has to be, "But why? Why would anyone want to even *joke* about subjecting our food supply to nuclear waste, let alone actually *do* it?" Ostensibly it is for your safety. People are deathly afraid of certain bacteria like salmonella, E. coli, Listeria and the like, which primarily infect animal products such as beef, pork, chicken and other meat. Relying on this fear, food irradiation of animal products was relatively easy to initiate. From that, for strictly financial reasons, it has been decided to irradiate *everything*. It is true that irradiation can kill most bacteria in food, but as is usually the case when something is being pulled off by those who will benefit while you will be harmed, some inconvenient facts are left out.

Conditions at most slaughterhouses and food-processing plants are already lax, and irradiation further masks and encourages filthy conditions. How? Because when bacterial contamination is held in check, a sense of complacency is the result. Yes, irradiation removes bacteria, but it does nothing to remove the feces, urine, pus and vomit that is often to be found.

Although there are numerous other serious factors of concern that the nuclear enthusiasts carefully exclude from their praise of food irradiation, let us turn to one that I find most alarming because of the extent to which it threatens your health and thereby your life. The proponents of food irradiation are quick to point out that it does not render food radioactive. That is true. However, it does render the food *dead*. The radiation doesn't only kill the bacteria, it also kills what's good in the food. How could it possibly be otherwise? You have certainly learned throughout this book about the incalculable value of enzymes. *All* life depends upon them. Once a food's enzymes are destroyed, it's dead. Irradiation kills enzymes, and that's not all it kills.

In discussing the effects of food irradiation, the FDA declared that *destruction of nutrients is not a concern*. For whom? It is fully acknowledged, even by the proponents of food irradiation, that it destroys nutrients, especially vitamins A, C, E, some Bs, essential fatty acids and other nutrients. In fact, the rationale employed to reconcile the use of nuclear waste to irradiate the *entire* food supply is that it's no different from the nutritional destruction that would result from cooking the food. Oh, great! Swell! That's terrific! If the premise of this book is correct, that we need to eat more living food and less cooked food in order to lose weight and improve health, and the irradiators have their way, there will be *only* cooked food available. *All* living food will be cooked, whether you like it or not. You will never again be able to eat a fresh piece of fruit or a fresh salad again. The FDA has already ruled that irradiated food *cannot* be labeled as fresh. Is that really what we need these days, *less* fresh food? Does your common sense resonate with that prospect?

Dear reader, even if what you have just learned about food irradiation rendering all living food lifeless was all there was to it, that would be *more* than enough reason to not irradiate our food. Living bodies *need* living food, and depriving our bodies of this primary essential of life can only lead to trouble. And even though precooking all of our food before we eat it is reason enough to ban food irradiation forevermore, there are a few other considerations that are equally troubling.

Don't ever forget that the nuclear industry is precisely that—an industry. It conducts business and makes money just like any other profit-based industry. Owing in large part to the moving away from nuclear proliferation, members of the nuclear industry have had to come up with new and innovative ways to boost their dwindling profits. In a desperate bid to do so, the unthinkable has been proposed. Aside from a nuclear bomb going off or some horrendous accident at a nuclear plant such as Chernobyl or Three Mile

Island, which releases radiation on the population, what is the most troublesome, menacing and perilous by-product of the nuclear industry? Nuclear waste! Disposing of the stuff has been a nonstop source of grief, aggravation and expense for the industry. We're talking about cesium 137 and cobalt 60, which are unimaginably toxic and deadly, and every effort to find a way to get rid of them is fraught with danger and opposition from people who don't want it anywhere near them. Dumping it in the ocean had environmentalists going ballistic. Burying it underground in Nevada, South Carolina and other places invariably incites people living near where it is buried to march in the streets and generally express their outrage. Plus it costs a lot of money to truck it across the country, bury it in an isolated site and guard it properly. A *lot* of money.

Oh, what to do, what to do! If only there was some need that could be created for nuclear waste, but what? Wouldn't it be great if, instead of *paying* millions of dollars to get rid of the stuff, there was a way to *make* millions of dollars by selling it? Goodness yes, but that would be just too much to hope for. Then in a stroke of sheer lunacy, a scheme, although far-fetched and improbable, was hatched.

Generally speaking, people have a fear of microorganisms such as germs and bacteria. In some instances it's justified; in some it's not. Obviously, salmonella and the like present a danger, but there are some germs and bacteria that are essential to life. In fact, if *all* germs and bacteria were to be destroyed, life would cease. Be that as it may, by and large, most people's attitude toward microorganisms is: Kill 'em.

The little bit of truth in many a lie is
what makes them so terrible.

—MARIE VON EBNER-ESCHENBACH

Considering that most people are terror-stricken at the thought of ingesting salmonella, E. coli, Listeria, mad cow disease or any number of other little nasties that like hanging around on decomposing animals, why not capitalize on that fear and parlay it into an industry? Since medical instruments were already being sterilized with radiation, the same process could be used on beef, chicken and pork so people could eat them without the fear of being struck down by some malevolent beastie lurking in their hamburgers. Slowly, over time, more and more foods could be radiated until every last morsel eaten by the American people would be subjected to irradiation. This would create an ongoing, nonstop need for nuclear waste. What was once a financial drain could be turned into a financial boon. With the proper "education," people could be taught to accept it as a viable solution to the contamination problem.

Beginning in 1986, the FDA has given the green light to expose nearly our entire food supply to nuclear irradiation. The only thing that has kept it from proliferating at a faster pace beyond animal products is the one giant snag the irradiators can't seem to overcome, and they won't overcome it unless they can figure out how to slip some potion into the water supply that successfully disengages people's common sense and natural inclination to *avoid nuclear waste!* It's a pesky problem.

The American people have already expressed a collective *no* to irradiated foods. Plus, over fifty years of scientific research documenting the dangers of irradiated food back that decision. According to a 1997 *CBS News* poll, 73 percent of people surveyed said that food should *not* be irradiated and 77 percent said they would not eat irradiated food, including 91 percent of women surveyed. Between 1998 and 2000, the percentage of shoppers who told the Food Marketing Institute that they would buy irradiated food dropped from 79 percent to 38 percent.

Did the proponents of the scheme listen? Heck, no. They're not going to allow a little thing like public opposition stop them from making billions of dollars while simultaneously finding a convenient and legal dumping ground for their troublesome nuclear waste: our food supply. The Department of Energy admitted as much when it stated to the House Armed Services Committee that, "The utilization of these radioactive materials simply reduces our waste handling problem." How nice for them. Instead of heeding citizen concerns, they came up with a better idea. Create what they refer to as a "consumer training" project designed to increase sales and enhance the image of irradiated foods. And guess who they determined should pay for this project? *You!* These people have no shame. Not only do they want to foist the most horrific and macabre scheme imaginable on an unsuspecting public, but they actually work it out so the public has to pay for the propaganda campaign that convinces them to like what they don't want. The very idea that the federal government would spend taxpayer dollars to promote a for-profit industry is objectionable, to say the least. But in order to promote the nuclear industry, which is in a panic to stay afloat, 600,000 of your taxpayer dollars are being spent to help them. The only beneficiaries of this campaign will be the large corporations involved in the irradiation industry, and *you* are footing the bill to get it launched. What is this, *Mad* magazine come to life?

As a side note, are you familiar with the International Atomic Energy Agency (IAEA)? In 1959, it was given the primary responsibility to research and develop nuclear technologies. The agency's board, which includes the United States, China and thirty-two other nations, has as one of its primary functions keeping nuclear arms out of the hands of countries like Iraq and North Korea. But here on the homefront they are the world's leading proponent of dousing your food with nuclear waste. Does it strike you as at all odd that the International Atomic Energy Agency, Department of Energy and Nuclear Regulatory Commission are making decisions about the condition of the food you and your family will eat?

Never have so many been
manipulated so much
by so few.

—ALDOUS HUXLEY

Let's get back to the "consumer training" project that you will be paying for to convince you to be more comfortable with having your food irradiated against your will, and not coincidentally, will also result in resuscitating the sagging nuclear industry. Now, since the goal and purpose of the project you were kind enough to fund against your wishes is to put you at ease over the entire issue, great care had to be taken to ensure that none of those annoying little truths are included, which might have the effect of turning you off. In keeping with that objective, the IAEA made its position crystal-clear. In one of its publications we find this little beauty: "We must confer with experts in the various fields of advertising and psychology to put the public at ease. Any word or statement containing the word 'radiation' or 'radiate' should not be required on the label." Gee, doesn't that make you feel all fuzzy and warm all over? They want to hire psychologists to figure out just the right word to use instead of the word that actually describes what is being attempted, so as to *trick* you into accepting this outrageous sham. Perhaps instead of calling it food irradiation, they could call it "food embracing" or "food kissing and hugging." That shouldn't offend anyone.

Actually, the most popular phrase being bandied about at present has to do with a word with which the public is already familiar. That way there would be acceptance by association. A completely meaningless, misleading and artificial euphemism is plucked right out of the air and delivered to your doorstep: "cold pasteurized" or "electronically pasteurized." Although consumers have rejected these phrases as deceptive and sneaky, the FDA has yet to rule them out. You must ask yourself why these people are going to such lengths to come up with phrases and descriptions designed specifically to keep you in the dark.

You should be apprised of another ploy that the nuclear industry uses to lull you into complacency, designed to desensitize you to the stark reality of actually using nuclear waste on the food supply. In addition to cesium 137 and cobalt 60, both of which are nuclear wastes, another means of radiating your food with ionizing radiation has been developed: "electronic beam," which is accomplished by what is referred to as a "linear accelerator." Note that these terms *specifically* refrain from mentioning the words "radiation" or "radiate," even though that's what is being done to the food.

Even though the linear accelerator radiates food and kills it to the same degree as cesium 137 and cobalt 60, it is not with a nuclear-waste product and therefore does not present the same environmental dangers. The plan is to get you accustomed to having your food destroyed by irradiation, and once you are comfortable with it (God forbid), the surplus cesium 137 and cobalt 60 can then be used—which is, after all, the true goal of this entire sham: to find a means to somehow dispose of nuclear waste. The linear accelerator is nothing more than a gimmick to distract you so the cesium 137 and cobalt 60 can be snuck in the back door.

Another objective of your "education" is one that is so laughable and outrageous that I can hardly write it without gagging. It is to increase your knowledge of the "wholesomeness of irradiated food." It is as though they are so arrogantly certain they can make a gullible public believe anything they want them to believe that they will say whatever they please no matter how absurd. If you deposited $10,000 in your bank account and were told by the bank that they "enriched" your account by crediting it with $2,000, would you feel enriched?

How by any stretch of the imagination could irradiated food be declared wholesome when animals fed irradiated foods in experiments dating back fifty years have suffered dozens of health problems, including premature death, mutations and other genetic abnormalities, fetal death and other reproductive problems, immune-system disorders, fatal internal bleeding, organ damage, tumors, stunted growth and nutritional deficiencies?

The folks yanking the wool over your eyes must not own a dictionary. If I'm not mistaken, the word "wholesome" probably comes from the word "whole." You know, complete, unfragmented, entirely intact. They openly admit that vitamins and other nutrients are destroyed, and that in their mind is wholesome. Alrighty then. Yet another objective is to convince you that irradiated food is safe. This is, of course, the biggie. Since we humans have somehow managed to survive for the last several hundred thousand years or so without the benefit of subjecting our food to radioactive nuclear waste, it's fairly certain that most people would prefer risking continuing to do so if there is even a *hint* of doubt as to the safety to irradiating food. My friends, there is one whole heck of a lot more than a hint.

You already know what my attitude is toward studies: Anyone can prove anything with the proper funding. True, there are some that are so flawlessly and impeccably conducted that their credibility and reliability are absolutely unimpeachable. And before I would subject myself and my loved ones to food treated with radioactive nuclear waste, I would insist on there being several hundred of the most highly regarded, unimpeachable studies ever conducted, wouldn't you? Anything less would be entirely unacceptable—end of conversation. I mean, why take a chance with something so very important just so the nuclear industry can get out of the red and show a profit?

How a report is framed, which
facts it contains and emphasizes, and
which it ignores and in what context are as
important to shaping opinion as
the bare facts themselves.

—MARK HERTSGAARD

The FDA reviewed 441 toxicity studies to determine the safety of irradiated foods. Dr. Marcia Gemert, the chairperson of the committee in charge of investigating the studies, testified that *all 441 were flawed*. In fact, the FDA claimed only 5 of the 441 were properly conducted. So let's see—with the shaky assurance of only five questionable studies, the FDA approved the use of irradiation from radioactive nuclear waste to be used on the entire public food supply. From this, proponents of food irradiation who stand to benefit the most from the decision want you to accept that it is safe.

Allow me to give you the nonfiction version.

Once again, I don't want to bog you down with a bunch of what-ifs, maybes and could-bes, although there are some well-educated guesses as to the problems that can result from messing around with nuclear waste, and they all are frightening. But let's just stick to the facts of what is already unquestionably known.

Radiation in the form of gamma rays emanating from radioactive cesium 137 or cobalt 60 is used to zap your food—enough gamma rays to easily kill a bystander several times over. If it is enough to kill a person, will it not do the same to your food?

Have you ever seen people going through a metal detector at an airport, taking a sandwich or some other food out of their bag and handing it to the guard because they didn't want it X-rayed? Are you hesitant to get a lot of dental or chest X rays? Generally, we have learned that the effects of X rays are cumulative in the body, so the fewer the better. And although one X ray here or there is probably not going to make a difference, the thinking is: the fewer, the better.

If you are the type of person described above who is concerned with the number of X rays you receive, you had better prepare yourself for what you are about to read. Picture this: You feel like having a healthy lunch, so you prepare a nice salad of several fresh ingredients that are bursting with all of the components that support life. But before eating the salad, you place it on a table in a closed room where not another living thing is to be found. Then, glowing radioactive rods of cobalt 60 are mechanically raised out of a pool of water, and the deadly rays of this agent of death bombard and deluge your salad for between a half hour and an hour, not with the equivalent of ten X rays —a hundred, a thousand or even a million—but with up to the equivalent of *tens of millions* of X rays' worth of radiation. It's hard to even fathom such astronomical numbers, isn't it? The rods are then lowered back into the water, and you put the salad in your mouth, chew it up and swallow it. That's millions of X rays on every bite of food you will ever eat, so you will never again eat a fresh or living food. What does your common sense tell you about that?

It is likely you have heard mention of free radicals and antioxidants. Oxygen is used by body cells to break down proteins, fats and carbohydrates, and in the process, free radicals are formed. Many authorities are convinced that free radicals are the precursor to cancer. All agree that free radicals are a danger to healthy cells. The body protects itself with compounds called antioxidants that either stop the formation of free radicals or disable them before they can do harm. Fruits and vegetables are, of course, brimming with antioxidants, which is one of the many reasons they are such an important part of a healthy diet and are universally recommended.

Using radioactive gamma rays to irradiate food breaks up the molecular structure of food and *forms* free radicals. These free radicals then react with the food to create new harmful chemical substances called "radiolytic products." And since they are unique to the irradiation process, they are commonly referred to as "unique radiolytic products." They are so common in irradiated food that they even have their own unique nickname: URPs. Knowing that free radicals are harmful and that antioxidants are beneficial, what does your common sense say about a process that *creates* more free radicals in your food while simultaneously *diminishing* its antioxidant content? Those pushing for this madness want you to think that such a process is wholesome. Some URPs such as formaldehyde, benzene, formic acid and quinones are known to be harmful to human health. There is one class of URP called cyclobutanones that do not occur naturally any where on Earth. Although they were first identified in irradiated foods in 1971, it was another *twenty-seven years* before German government scientists discovered that one type (there are several) caused genetic and cellular damage in humans. It took *twenty-seven years* to figure this out in only one of the many URPs that exist. There are some URPs that have not even been identified, let alone tested for toxicity. Should we not wait, just in case it takes twenty-seven years to determine the effect of some of the other URPs?

This is a form of Russian roulette with the highest stakes of all: your life. This area is a complete unknown in human experience. The only way we will ever find out for sure if irradiated food is safe is to wait twenty or thirty years when the results of its consumption can be viewed. So the people who are willing now to be the guinea pigs in this experiment will tell the story for those who follow. Want to volunteer? Want to volunteer your children? Are you willing to throw the dice with your family's life on the line and hope for the best? We're not talking about something benign; we're talking about *nuclear waste!* What does your common sense tell you about that?

There is one last consideration to contemplate if the nuclear enthusiasts get their way and *all* food is irradiated. Where do you think all of this irradiating is going to take place? Do you think it will be far from your home in some isolated part of the world? In the desert or in the Arctic, or some other faraway place? It will take place in the cities or towns where you are presently living, that's where.

The essence of propaganda is the presentation of one side of the picture only.

—J. A. C. BROWN

Supporters of food irradiation often say that irradiation facilities are safe. They say accidents rarely happen. They say injuries and death are infrequent. They say the public is in no danger. The historical record says otherwise. Since the 1960s, dozens of accidents, as well as numerous acts of wrongdoing, have been reported at irradiation facilities throughout the United States. Radioactive water has been flushed down toilets into the public sewer system. Radioactive waste has been thrown into the garbage. Radiation has leaked. Facilities have caught fire. Equipment has malfunctioned. Workers have lost fingers, hands, legs and, in several cases, their lives. Company executives have been charged with cover-ups and, in one case, sentenced to federal prison.

In Decatur, Georgia, in June 1988 there was a leak of cesium 137 that resulted in a $30 million cleanup that the taxpayers had to pay. In Dover, New Jersey, two senior executives of an irradiation plant were indicted on federal charges of conspiracy, mail fraud and wire fraud after a 1982 spill of radioactive cobalt 60 that workers were instructed to pour down a shower drain into the public sewer system. In Honolulu in 1979 a plant was shut down after radioactive water leaked onto the roof and the front lawn. New Jersey is home to the highest concentration of irradiation facilities, and virtually every one has a record of environmental contamination, worker overexposure or regulatory failures. There are so many more accidents I could tell you about that are not only problematic for the workers, but to the surrounding communities as well. *Your* community.

With only about fifty irradiation facilities in the United States, the NRC has its hands full trying to cope with and keep in check all the problems at all the sites. If this ill-conceived plan to irradiate the *entire* food supply comes to pass, there won't be fifty nuclear-waste sites; there will be more like a *thousand*. That's a twentyfold increase, an average of twenty for every state in the country. What state do you live in? How close are you willing to allow one of the twenty in *your* state to be to your home? You wouldn't mind having your kids play only a stone's throw from one, would you? Instead of a few central locations where nuclear waste is buried underground, there will be thousands of trucks and trains traveling the highways and railway lines to every town and city in the country. How long will it be before the first catastrophe occurs, which will cause people to rethink the idea after it's too late?

Irrespective of the devastating effect on our health that will occur as a result of not being able to obtain any living food, there is yet another consideration for which we have no choice but to ponder. We are living at a very tumultuous and unpredictable time in history. There are murderous madmen—Osama bin Laden and his ilk—skulking around, looking for any opportunity to harm the United States and its people. Do we really want to construct a *thousand* nuclear-waste sites spread out all over the country for them to target? They must be licking their chops at the prospect. Shall we take such a risk in order to bring to market *less wholesome food?* Aside from the financial benefit that will accrue to the nuclear industry, where's the upside?

Throughout this book I have pointed out numerous cashectomies—the process of selling you something with the promise of all the good it will do you but giving you instead something that harms or kills you. The attempt to use radioactive nuclear waste on the food supply under the guise of its being healthy, wholesome and safe has to be the most sinister scheme ever conjured up in the devil's workshop. It is not merely a cashectomy; it is a cashectomy squared.

There is a question I would like to ask you, and with a matter of such importance as this, it is a question you should ask yourself. If nuclear waste were not available to be used in this scheme, do you think for one moment there would be anyone trying to figure out how to irradiate our food? If nuclear waste did not exist, could you imagine someone in a think tank set up to figure out ways of improving the quality of life suggesting that some waste from nuclear reactors be used to treat the entire food supply? Such a suggestion would be met with the same enthusiasm that would greet the suggestion that everyone take out a rusty ice pick and plunge it into his or her eyeball.

Of all the hard things to bear and grin, the hardest of all is being taken in.

—Phoebe Cary

If there were not tons of cesium 137 and cobalt 60 lying around presenting the problem of disposal, food irradiation would not even be a subject of discussion. That's because food irradiation is not the true goal. This entire thing is about finding a means to get rid of nuclear garbage and reviving the floundering nuclear industry. If you knew *nothing* whatsoever about this subject, not one thing, and someone were to stop you on the street and ask you if you would like to have your food treated with radioactive nuclear waste before eating it, what do you think your instantaneous, instinctive response would be? What would your common sense dictate? Let *that* rule your thinking on this issue, not the propaganda of the power brokers.

When I was a young boy in the mid-1950s, I lived in the small coal-mining town of Harlan, Kentucky. It was one of those small towns where everyone knew everyone else and looked after one another. So on the weekends it was perfectly safe for my folks to drop me off at a movie theater and pick me up a few hours later. I would be given twenty-five cents, which was enough to pay for admission, a bag of popcorn and a soda. (Today twenty-five cents won't even pay for two Raisinets.)

Aside from the feeling of freedom I experienced at being "on my own," so to speak, even though I was only seven or eight years old, what is most indelibly sealed in my memory is the thick, foul air that always hung in the auditorium. You see, in those days, anyone—anywhere, at any time—could light up and smoke a cigarette, cigar or pipe. My eyes would sting and my clothes would smell foul, but that's just the way it was. There were no smoking and non-smoking sections; the entire world and every place in it was the smoking section. It was the same on airplanes. Every armrest had its own ashtray, no matter where you sat on the plane.

Don't think there weren't people at the time who were adamantly opposed to smoking in public places, because there were. They would talk of the dire consequences thirty or forty years down the line if the habit were not banned, but they were effectively silenced by the power brokers of that era. Dissenters were labeled as health nuts, crackpots or busybodies trying to spoil it for everyone. Besides, everyone knew smoking was harmless; it was even advertised by doctors in magazines or on that newfangled invention called the television. Medical doctors would come on and extol the virtues of one brand or another. The American Medical Association even owned millions of dollars of tobacco stocks. Consider the following statement made by Ian G. MacDonald, M.D.: "Cigarette smoking is a harmless pastime up to twenty-four cigarettes a day. One could modify an old slogan: A pack a day keeps lung cancer away."

Yes! He actually said those very words. And he wasn't some doctor-for-hire, shilling for the tobacco industry. He was the chairman of the Committee on Cancer Research at the American Medical Association. And he wasn't uttering these pearls of wisdom in a drunken stupor at a backyard barbecue. They are part of the official record because he made the statements before the Subcommittee on Legal and Monetary Affairs at the House Government Operations Committee on July 25, 1957. Now that we know that more than 1,250 people die every day (469,000 a year) in the United States because of smoking, it's easy to look back fifty years later and lament that we didn't listen to the "crackpots" and save all those lives.

History teaches us the mistakes
we are going to make.

—LAURENCE J. PETER

It's not tragic to make a mistake; it's human. What is tragic is when we fail to learn from our mistakes and make the same ones over again. We have a chance right now to not make one of the greatest blunders history will ever record. Thirty or forty or fifty years from now, a student in school somewhere will write a report about the concept born in the last part of the twentieth century to irradiate the food supply with radioactive nuclear waste. Whether that report will focus on what a tragic and deadly mistake was made or on how close we came to making it is up to you right now. Will you listen to today's dissenters or to those with a vested interest? Will we find out forty years too late that lives could have been saved and a tragedy averted, as would have been the case if smoking was discouraged earlier on?

History has shown us over and over that those who have enormous wealth and therefore wield immense power and influence have consistently gotten their way. It is rare indeed when the so-called "little people" are victorious when going to battle against the rich and powerful. Not that it hasn't happened, because it has. One can only wonder how long the Vietnam War would have raged on were it not for like-minded and committed Americans who *demanded* that it end. They marched in the streets and would not be silenced. It was the same with the civil rights marches of the 1960s. Blacks and whites marched hand-in-hand and put their lives on the line in order to bring about change. Huge numbers of people acting in unison are more powerful than any group, no matter how much money and how much influence they possess.

Although the nuclear industry and those who support it do have unimaginable resources at their command and are willing to do whatever it takes to get what they want, there is one ingredient in the equation they absolutely *must* have, and without which they are completely impotent. Guess what that ingredient is? *You!* If you are not willing to spend your money on irradiated food, the entire fiasco is dead in the water. They need to have your cooperation. It's a sad commentary, I know, but this entire thing is about money, and if you're not willing to spend it—case closed.

You must be convinced to accept and participate in food irradiation. That is precisely why, even though people's common sense and instincts have caused them to reject it, a $600,000 "consumer education and training" project is necessary to convince you that it is "safe and wholesome," even though the facts prove otherwise.

This is not an issue to put on the back burner of your priorities. This is not something you should leave up to others. I'm not asking you to write to Congress or to march in the streets, but I am asking you to make your feelings known where you spend your food dollars. When you are in the grocery store, take the time to ask which foods have been irradiated because you don't want them and won't buy them. You will then quickly learn who has the *real* power, and this atrocious fiasco can be put to rest.

* * * * * *

There are several organizations that have been fighting for your rights on this issue for decades. They are committed and tireless, and we owe them a great debt of gratitude for their efforts in keeping the nuclear industry at bay for as long as they have. I obtained the particular facts and figures I have written about here from them, and you can (and should) contact them to learn more.

The one I am most familiar with and have been in communication with for twenty years is:

Food & Water, Inc.
Post Office Box #543
Montpelier, VT 05601
800-EAT-SAFE
www.foodandwater.com

Two other very important groups are:

Public Citizen
215 Pennsylvania Ave., S.E.
Washington, DC 20003
202-546-4996
www.citizen.org/cmep

GRACE
215 Lexington Ave., Suite #1001
New York, NY 10016
212-726-9161
www.gracelinks.org

CHAPTER NOTES

Introduction

1. Geoffrey Cowley, "Generation XXL," *Newsweek*, July 3, 2000.

Chapter 1

1. "Heavyweight Solutions," Discovery Health Channel, Sept. 8, 2002.

2. Emma Ross, "World Health Organization Toughening Approach to Obesity Battle," Associated Press, May 29, 2002.

3. George Gurdjieff, *All and Everything* (New York: E. P. Dutton & Co., 1950).

4. "Study: 2 Million Get Sick from Drugs," *Washington Post*, Apr. 15, 1998.

5. Sheryl Gay Stolberg, "Officials: Risk from Medicine Growing," *New York Times*, June 3, 1999.

6. Op. cit., chapter 1, note 2.

7. "Clinical Guidelines on the Identification, Evaluation and Treatment of Overweight and Obesity in Adults," National Institutes of Health, vol. 6, supplement 2, 1998.

8. A. H. Mokdad, M. K. Serdula, W. H. Dietz, et al., "The Spread of the Obesity Epidemic in the United States," *Journal of the American Medical Association* 282.16 (1999).

9. Op. cit., chapter 1, note 2.

10. "Study Says Obesity Causes 90,000 Cancer Deaths Each Year," The Associated Press, Apr. 24, 2003.

11. Ibid.

12. R. P. Troiano, K. M. Flegal, "Overweight Children and Adolescents: Description, Epidemiology and Demographics," *Pediatrics* 101 (1998).

13. "Stomach Hormone May Be Key to Long-Term Weight Loss," *Washington Post*, May 23, 2002.

Chapter 2

1. Ian Anderson, "Stages of Life," *The Incredible Machine* (Washington, D.C.: National Geographic Society, 1986).

2. *New England Journal of Medicine*, Oct. 24, 1985.

3. Francis M. Pottenger, "The Effect of Heat-Processed Foods and Metabolized Vitamin D Milk on the Dentofacial Structures of Experimental Animals," *American Journal of Orthodontics and Oral Surgery* 8, Aug. 1946.

4. Edmond B. Szekely, *The Essene Gospel of Peace* (United States: International Biogenic Society, 1981).

Chapter 5

1. Herbert M. Shelton, *The Hygienic Care of Children* (Bridgeport, Conn.: Natural Hygiene Press, 1981).

2. Hillary Ferrara, "Raw Energy," *Sarasota Herald Tribune*, Sept. 4, 2002.

3. A. C. Guyton, M.D., *Medical Physiology* (New York: W. B. Saunders, 1962).

4. Herbert M. Shelton, "Natural Hygiene: Man's Pristine Way of Life," Dr. Shelton's Health School, Texas, 1968.

5. James M. Rippe, *Dr. James M. Rippe's Complete Book of Fitness Walking* (New York: Prentice Hall, 1989).

Chapter 6

1. Op. cit., chapter 2, note 4.

Chapter 7

1. "Most Weight Loss Ads Are Deceptive, FTC Study Says," Associated Press, Sept. 18, 2002.

2. Paul Jacobs, "Near Miracles and Mental States," *Los Angeles Times*, Mar. 18, 1984.

3. Harvey Diamond, *The Fit for Life Solution* (St. Paul, Minn.: Dragon Door Publishers, 2002).

4. Steven Findlay, "Pain Is Our #1 Health Complaint," *USA Today*, Oct. 23, 1985.

5. "United States Health Care Tab Soars to $1.3 Trillion," *Health Freedom News*, Apr./May 2002.

6. "The Dismal Truth About Teenage Health," *Reader's Digest*, Mar. 1986.

7. Marlene Simons, "U.S. Urges Cholesterol Cut Even If Disease Risk Is Low," *Los Angeles Times*, Feb. 28, 1990.

8. G. Fraser, "The Effects of Various Vegetable Supplements on Serum Cholesterol," *American Journal of Clinical Nutrition* 34, 1981.

9. "Fiber Study: Supplement Might Harm the Colon," Associated Press, Oct. 13, 2000.

10. Tom Regan, "But for the Sake of Some Little Mouthful of Flesh," *The Animal's Agenda*, Feb. 1989.

Agriculture Statistics, 1988, U.S. Department of Agriculture.

11. Ibid.

12. Robin Hur, "Six Inches from Starvation: How and Why America's Topsoil Is Disappearing," *Vegetarian Times*, Mar. 1985.

David Pimental, et al., "Land Degradation: Effects on Food and Energy," *Science* 194, Oct. 1976.

National Association of Conservation Districts, Washington, D.C., "Soil Degradation: Effects on Agricultural Productivity," Interim Report #4, National Agricultural Land Study, 1980.

Seth King, "Farms Go Down the River," *New York Times*, Dec. 10, 1978.

13. David Pimental, et al., *Advances in Food Research*, vol. 32 (Academic Press: 1988).

14. *Statistical Abstract of the United States*. Exhibits #1211 and 1221, 1982–83.

Soil and Water Resources Conservation Act, review draft part I, appraisal 1980, U.S. Department of Agriculture.

15. National Agriculture Land Study, National Resources Inventory, 1982.

Agricultural Statistics, U.S. Department of Agriculture, 1981 and 1988.

Op. cit., chapter 7, note 13.

16. Mary Bralove, "The Food Crisis: The Shortages May Pit the 'Have Nots' Against the 'Haves,'" *Wall Street Journal*, Oct. 3, 1974.

Agricultural Statistics, U.S. Department of Agriculture, 1984.

17. Robin Hur and David Fields, Ph.D., "Are High-Fat Diets Killing Our Forests?" *Vegetarian Times*, Feb. 1984.

18. Frances Moore Lappe, *Diet for a Small Planet*, 10th ann. ed. (New York: Ballantine Books, 1982).

Alan Durning, Worldwatch Institute researcher.

19. "The Browning of America," *Newsweek*, Feb. 22, 1981.

20. Georg Borgstrom, presentation to the annual meeting of the American Association for the Advancement of Science.

Paul and Anne Ehrlich, *Population, Resources, Environment* (New York: W. H. Freeman, 1972).

21. *Soil and Water Resources Conservation Act*, 1980 appraisal review draft, part I, U.S. Department of Agriculture.

Georg Borgstrom, cited in *Diet for a Small Planet*, 1975 ed.

Raymond Loehr, "Pollution Implications of Animal Wastes," *Water Pollution Control Research* series, Washington, D.C., Office of Research Monitoring, U.S. Environmental Protection Agency, 1968.

22. Jim Mason and Pete Singer, *Animal Factories* (New York: Crown Publishers, 1980).

David Pimental, "Energy and Land Constraints in Food Protein Production," *Science*, Nov. 21, 1975.

H. A. Jasiorowski, "Intensive Systems of Animal Production," *Proceedings of the Third World Conference on Animal Production*, R. F. Reid, ed. (Sydney: Sydney University Press, 1975).

Jackie Robbins, "Environmental Impact Resulting from Unconfined Animal Production," *Environmental Protection Technology* series, U.S. Environmental Protection Agency, Office of Research and Development, Environmental Research Information Center, Cincinnati, Ohio, Feb. 1978.

23. Bruce Myles, "U.S. Antipollution Laws May Boost Cattle Feeders' Costs and Meat Prices," *Christian Science Monitor*, Mar. 11, 1974.

24. *Commercial Fertilizer Consumption in the United States*, U.S. Department of Agriculture, Statistical Reporting Service, 1985.

25. Statistical Abstract of the United States, 103rd ed., 1982–83, U.S. Department of Commerce, Bureau of Census, table #344.

26. Op. cit., chapter 7, note 21.

27. Robin Hur and David Fields, "How Meat Robs America of Its Energy," *Vegetarian Times*, Apr. 1985.

J. T. Reid, "Comparative Efficiency of Animals in the Conversion of Feedstuffs to Human Foods," *Confinement*, Apr. 1976.

W. L. Roller, et al., "Energy Costs of Intensive Livestock Production," American Society of Agricultural Engineers, June 1975, St. Joseph, Michigan, paper #75-4042, table #7.

[AUTHOR'S NOTE: Research for chapter 7, note 27 was done by Robin Hur. Information was garnered from a vast number of government organizations and private trade organizations. Some notable ones were the National Agricultural Land Study; U.S. Department of Agriculture; U.S. Department of Energy; U.S. Department of Transportation; Bureau of Economic Analysis; Bureau of the Census; Federal Highway Administration; Oak Ridge National Laboratories.]

28. William Brune, state conservationist, Soil Conservation Service, Des Moines, Iowa: Testimony before Senate Committee on Agriculture and Forestry, July 6, 1976.

Seth King, "Iowa Rain and Wind Deplete Farm Lands," *New York Times*, Dec. 5, 1976.

Curtis Harnack, "In Plymouth County, Iowa, the Rich Topsoil's Going Fast, Alas," *New York Times*, July 11, 1980.

29. Op. cit., chapter 7, note 10.

30. "World Hunger," report by the Food and Agricultural Organization of the United Nations (FAO), Rome, Italy, fall 1989.

Lester Brown, [of] The Overseas Development Council, as cited in "Diet for a New America," 1987.

Chapter 9

1. "Prilosec Might Be Sold Without Prescription," Associated Press, June 22, 2002.

2. R. Stein, "High Blood Pressure Rising," *Washington Post*, July 9, 2003.

Chapter 10

1. T. Osborn, "Amino Acids in Nutrition and Growth," *Journal of Biological Chemistry* 17, 1914.

2. T. Colin Campbell, M.D., et al., *Cornell–Oxford–China Project on Nutrition, Health and Environment, Diet, Lifestyle and Mortality in China: A Study of the Characteristics of Sixty-Five Countries* (Oxford: Oxford University Press, The China People's Medical Publishing House, 1990).

3. "Huge Study of Diet Indicts Fat and Meats," *New York Times*, May 8, 1990.

4. Lindsey H. Allen, Ph.D., et al., "Protein-Induced Hypercalcuria: A Long-Term Study," *American Journal of Clinical Nutrition*, Apr. 1979.

Chander R. Anand, et al., "Effect of Protein Intake on Calcium Balance of Young Men Given 500 Milligrams of Calcium Daily," *Journal of Nutrition*, Jan./June 1974.

Elaine Blume, "Protein," *Nutrition Action*, Mar. 1987.

"The Case Against Meat and Dairy," *Nutrition Health Review*, July 1985.

J. H. Cummings, et al., "The Effect of Meat Protein and Dietary Fiber on Colonic Function and Metabolism, Changes in Bowel Habits, Bile Acid Excretion and Calcium Absorption," *American Journal of Clinical Nutrition*, Oct. 1979.

Nan K. Fuchs, Ph.D., *The Nutrition Detective* (Los Angeles: J. P. Tarcher, 1985).

D. M. Hegsted, "Calcium and Osteoporosis," *Journal of Nutrition*, Nov. 1986.

Maren Hegsted, et al., "Urinary Calcium and Calcium Balance in Young Men as Affected by Level of Protein and Phosphorous Intake," *Journal of Nutrition*, Jan./June 1981.

Nancy E. Johnson, et al., "Effect of Level of Protein Intake on Urinary and Fecal Calcium and Calcium Retention of Young Adult Males," *Journal of Nutrition*, July/Dec. 1970.

H. Linkswiler, "Calcium Retention of Young Adult Males as Affected by Level of Protein and of Calcium Intake," *Transcript of New York Academy of Science* 36, 1974.

Helen M. Linkswiler, *Nutrition Review's Present Knowledge in Nutrition*, 4th ed. (New York: The Nutrition Foundation, 1976).

S. Margen, M.D., et al., "Studies in Calcium Metabolism, the Calciuretic Effect of Dietary Protein," *American Journal of Clinical Nutrition*, June 1974.

John A. McDougall, M.D., *McDougall's Medicine* (Secaucus, N. J.: New Century Publishers, 1985).

John A. McDougall, M.D., *McDougall's Plan* (Secaucus, N.J.: New Century Publishers, 1983).

Ammon Wachman, M.D., and Daniel B. Bernstein, M.D., "Diet and Osteoporosis," *Lancet*, May 4, 1968.

Ruth M. Walker, et al., "Calcium Retention in the Adult Human Male as Affected by Protein Intake," *Journal of Nutrition*, July/Dec. 1972.

Julian M. Whitaker, M.D., *Reversing Heart Disease* (New York: Warner Books, 1985).

5. Robin Hur, *Food Reform: Our Desperate Need* (Austin, Tex.: Heidelberg Publications, 1975).

6. Ibid.

7. George E. Lewinnek, M.D., "The Significance and a Comparative Analysis of the Epidemiology of Hip Fractures," *Clinical Orthopedics and Related Research*, Oct. 1980.

United Nations Food and Agricultural Organization, *FAO Production Yearbook*, 37, 1984.

United Nations Food and Agricultural Organization, *Food Balance Sheets: 1979–81 Average* (Rome, Italy, 1984).

Alexander R. P. Walker, D.Sc., "The Human Requirement of Calcium: Should Low Intakes Be Supplemented?" *American Journal of Clinical Nutrition*, May 1972.

Alexander R. P. Walker, D.Sc., "Osteoporosis and Calcium Deficiency," *Journal of Clinical Nutrition*, Mar. 1965.

8. Ibid.

9. Ibid.

10. Op. cit., chapter 10, note 3.

11. "Surgery for Obese Kids Gains Popularity," Associated Press, Nov. 6, 2002.

12. *Lancet*, Jan. 1960, p. 230.

13. Matt Crenson, "Yes We Have No Bananas—But Pass the Fries," Associated Press, Nov. 10, 2002.

14. Maureen Kennedy Salaman, "Suffer the Little Children, Processed Food Is Maiming Them," *Health Freedom News*, Oct./Nov. 2002.

15. "Drug Industry on a $125 Billion Roll," *Health Freedom News*, Jan./Feb. 2001.

16. Theresa Agovino, "Prescription Drugs' Growth Market: Kids," Associated Press, Sept. 19, 2002.

17. Op. cit., chapter 10, note 15.

18. "Rash of New Drugs Shot in Arm for Prescription Sales," Associated Press, Aug. 31, 1998.

19. Op. cit., chapter 10, note 16.

20. Op. cit., chapter 10, note 14.

21. Ibid.

22. "Push to Test Medicines on Children Overturned," Associated Press, Oct. 19, 2002.

23. Adam Liptak, "Plaintiff Suing over Free Prozac Sent in Mail," *New York Times*, July 6, 2002.

24. Op. cit., chapter 10, note 14.

25. Monroe E. Burton, "The Limbic Brain," *Acres, U.S.A.*, Feb. 1987.

26. Mary Georger, Center for Cardiovascular Research at the University of Rochester, Oct. 2002.

27. J. P. Koplan, et al., "Physical Activity, Physical Fitness and Health: Time to Act," *Journal of American Medical Association*, Nov. 3, 1991.

28. C. Wiley, "Walk This Way," *Vegetarian Times*, Jan. 1992.

29. Op. cit., chapter 10, note 27.

30. Op. cit., chapter 5, note 5.

31. Ibid.

32. Ibid.

33. Ibid.

34. Ibid.

35. B. Hottinger, "Walking Your Way to Fitness," *Vegetarian Voice,* vol. 18, no. 4.

36. Op. cit., chapter 5, note 5; chapter 10, notes 28 and 35.

37. University of California, Berkeley, *Wellness Letter.*

The Wellness Encyclopedia (Boston: Houghton Mifflin, 1991).

38. Op. cit., chapter 10, note 28.

39. Phillip N. Norman, M.D., "Food Combinations: An Original Scheme of Eating Based upon the Newer Knowledge of Nutrition and Digestion," 21, Sept. 12, 1924.

40. Martin Katahn, Ph.D., *The T-Factor Diet* (New York: Bantam Books, 1989).

41. *CBS News* with Dan Rather, June 6, 2002.

42. Ibid.

INDEX

ABOUT THE AUTHOR

Harvey Diamond has dedicated thirty-plus years of his life to the development of a truly healthy lifestyle. In pursuit of that goal, he overcame a debilitating, longtime digestive disorder, ended his migraine headaches, lost over fifty pounds, and in a stunning validation of his methods, triumphed over a condition called peripheral neuropathy (brought about by Agent Orange poisoning while serving his country in Vietnam).

Harvey's first *Fit for Life* book held the number-one position on the *New York Times* bestseller list for an unprecedented forty straight weeks and has sold over 12 million copies worldwide, where it is read in thirty-three languages in more than seventy countries.

One of the world's most dynamic and motivating authors and speakers, Harvey has the unusual ability to entertain while he educates. He calls it "edu-tainment." His down-to-earth, nontechnical, common-sense approach to well-being manages to enroll all who read his books or hear him speak, regardless of age, gender, education, profession, cultural background or interest. With unfailing good humor, he succeeds in sharing his considerable knowledge of health and nutrition and their effects on the human body in a way that makes his audiences *want* to try his recommendations. He shares your concerns and is able to clear up confusion on what is frequently a complicated subject, while offering easily attainable goals for everyone. Each person is left with the knowledge of what can be done to ensure a healthier, longer life starting that very day. He does all this and leaves you laughing.

His witty, knowledgeable and passionate words have given millions of people real hope and invaluable information to live life in what he calls "our God-given right of vibrant health." His energy, charisma and relaxed, conversational style have made him a sought-after guest expert on countless radio and television shows, including *Oprah*, *Geraldo*, *Nightline*, *Larry King Live*, *Live with Regis*, *The Today Show* and many others.

A MESSAGE FROM THE AUTHOR

Perhaps you are familiar with the phrase, "Often imitated—never duplicated." The name *Fit for Life* was coined for the ideas and book I cowrote in 1985. Over the years, as *Fit for Life* gained notoriety, the name has been used by a number of entities with which I have no personal connection.

I would like to assure you of my continued interest in hearing from you with any questions, comments or experiences you may have as a result of reading this book.

In addition, to order or obtain more information about products, services or my newsletter, the official contact points for me are as follows:

Postal address:

Harvey Diamond

P.O. Box 811

Osprey, Florida 34229

Web site:
www.fitforlifetime.com

E-mail:
info@fitforlifetime.com

Fax:
305-723-6166

Products:
Live Plant Enzymes; water; coral calcium; REBOUND*AIR*
rebounder; Teeter inversion table;
or for information or a catalog on the full line
of Feeling Fit products,
call toll free:
877-942-4492 or 877-215-1212

Speaking engagements/seminars:
941-966-1509